Hip Surgeries

Edited by Nahum Rosenberg

Published in London, United Kingdom

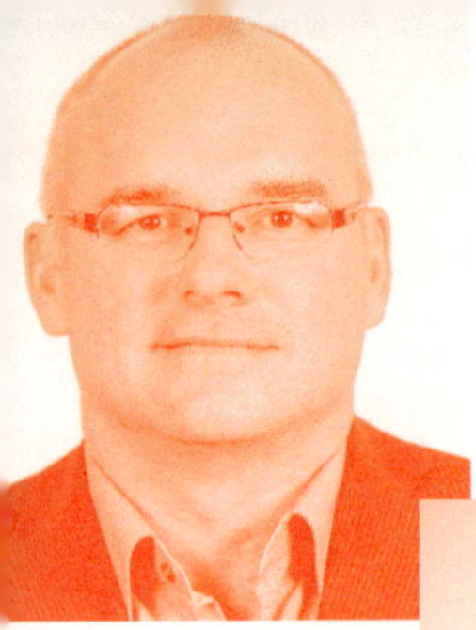
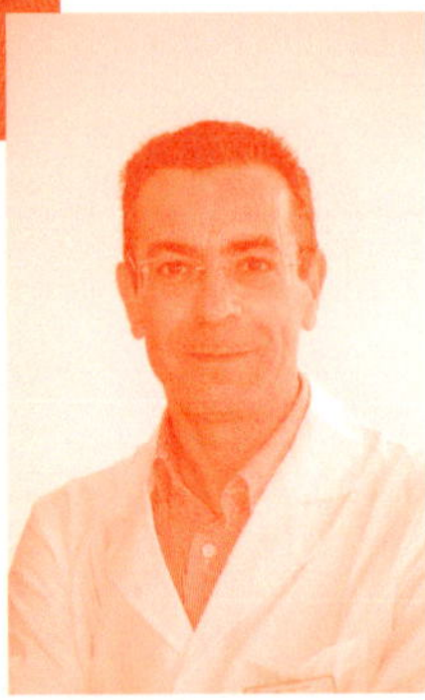
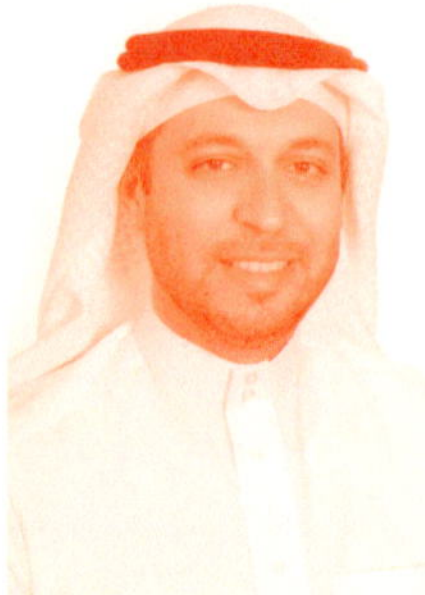
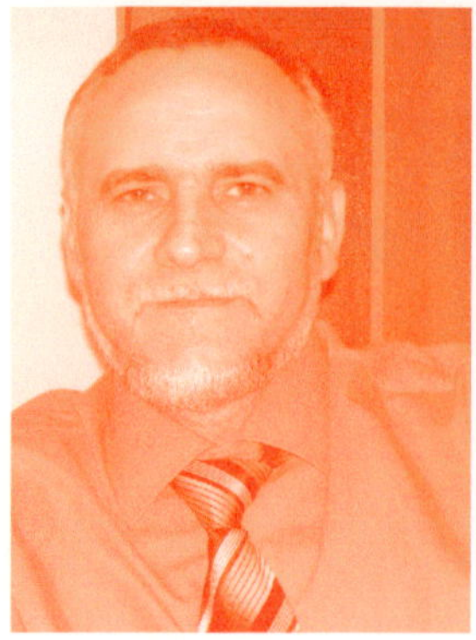
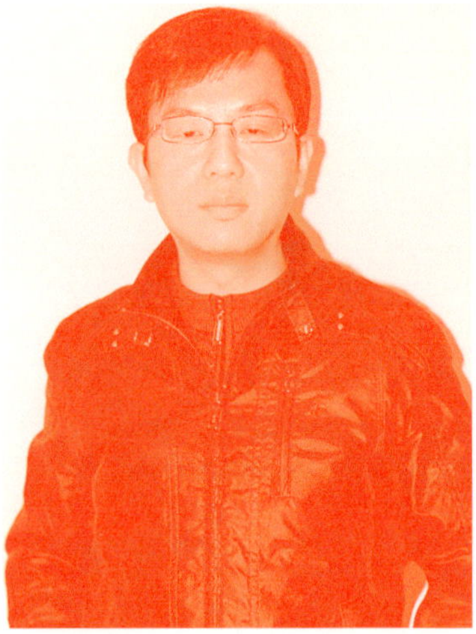
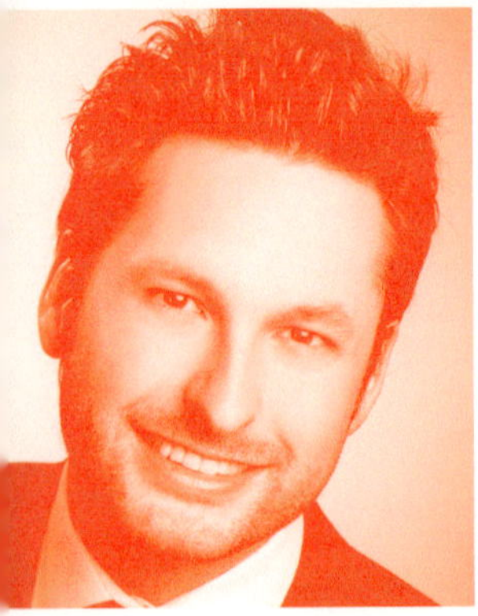
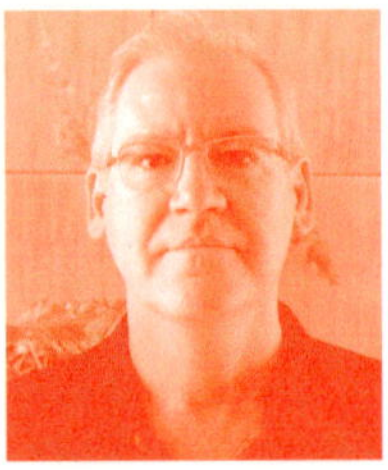

IntechOpen

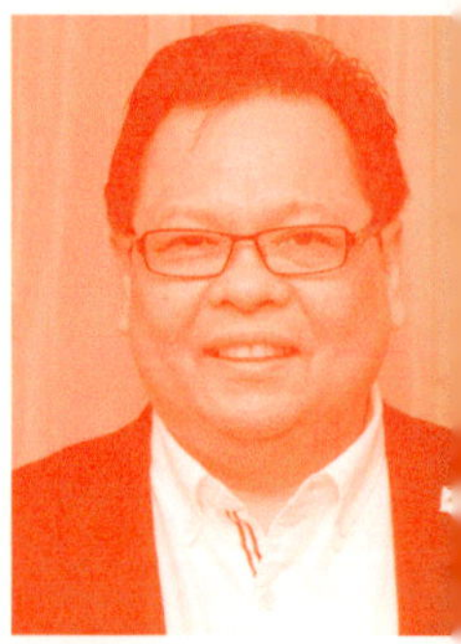
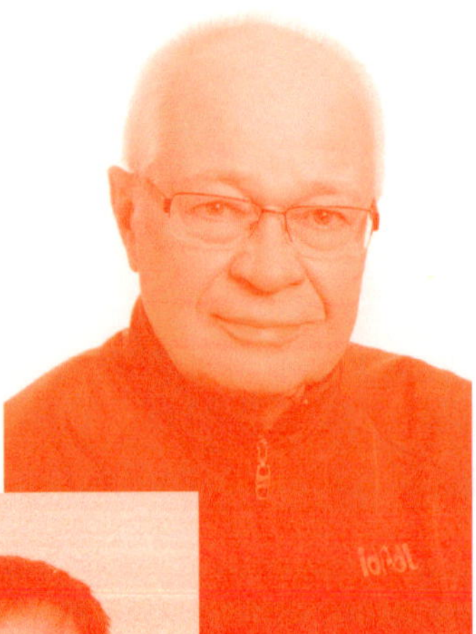
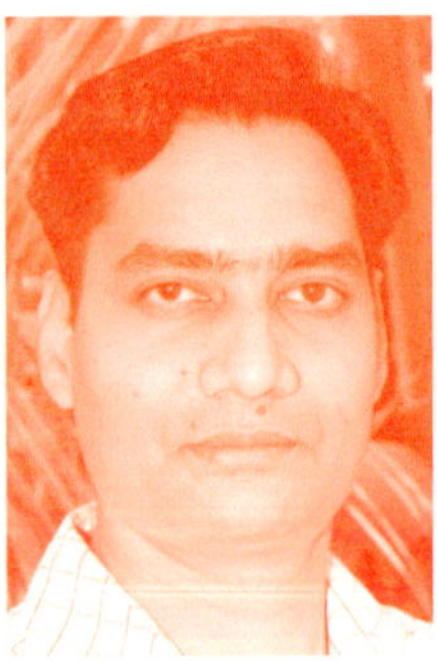
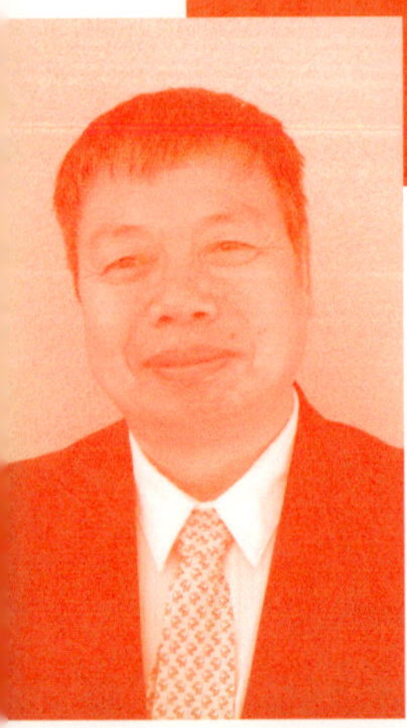
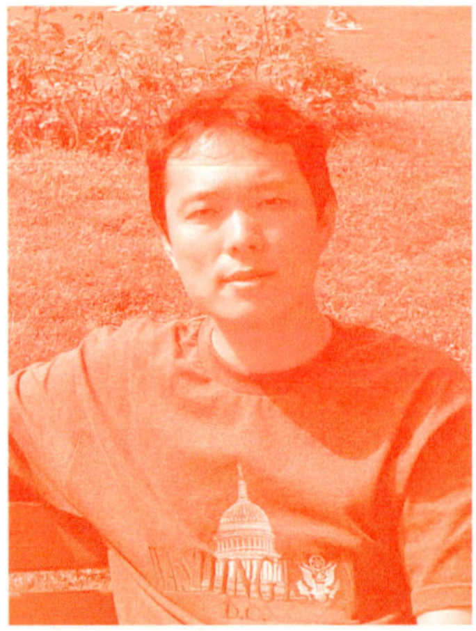
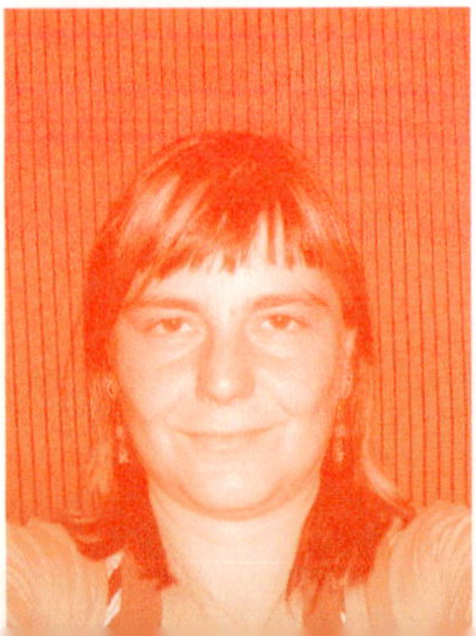

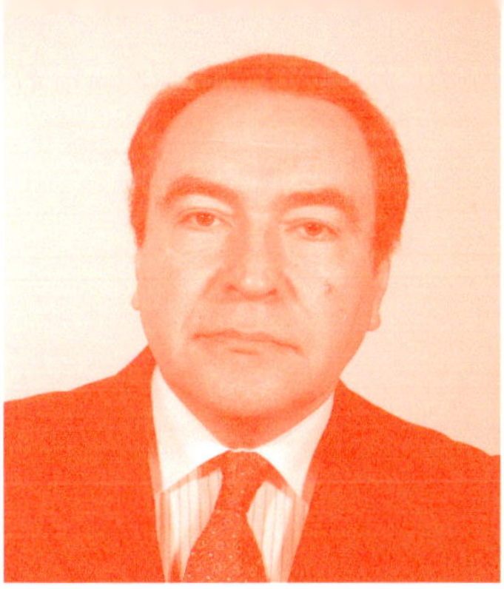
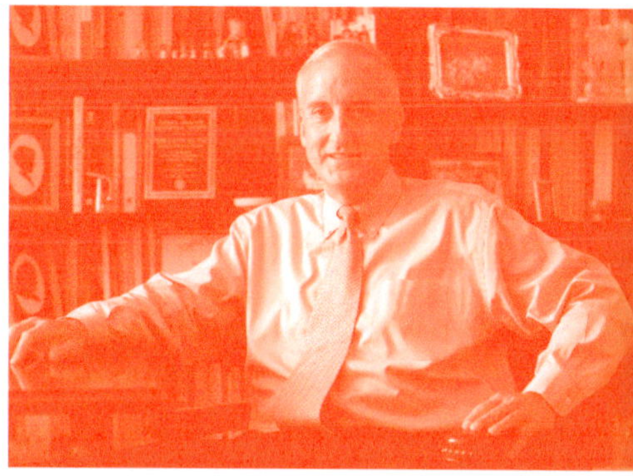
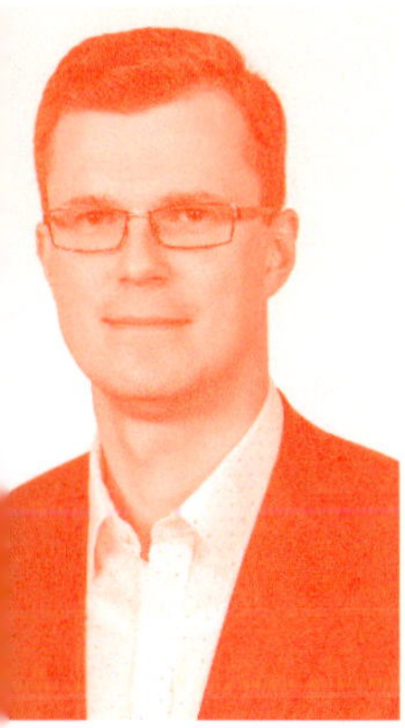
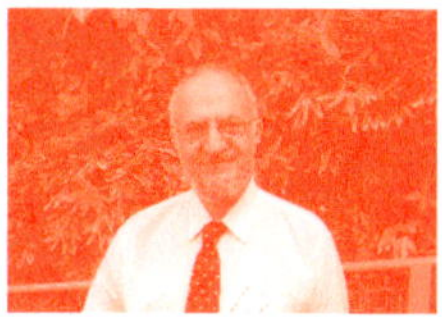
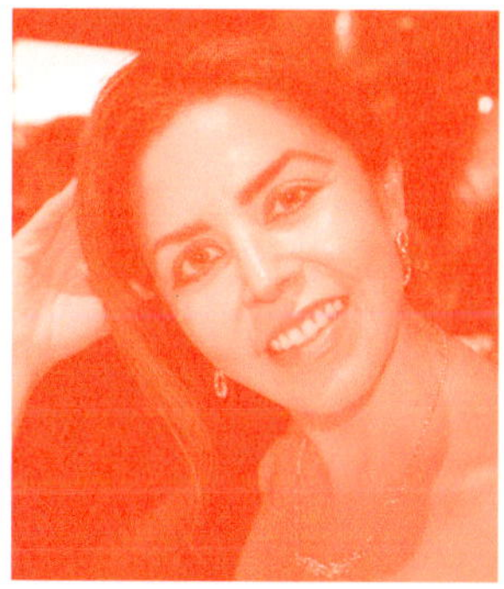

Supporting open minds since 2005

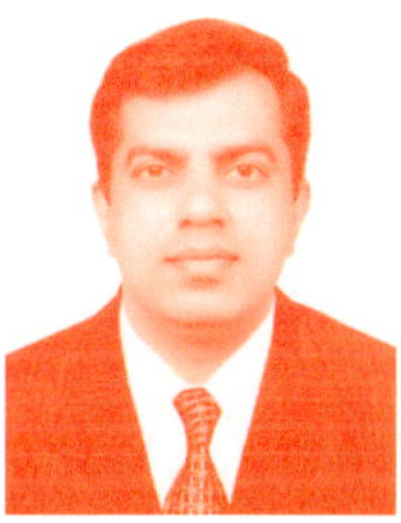
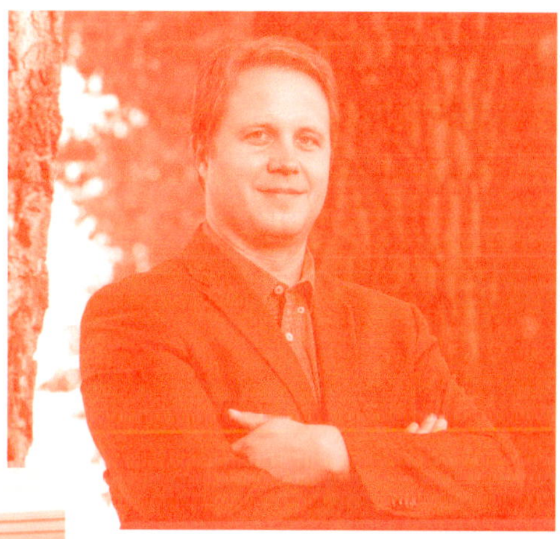
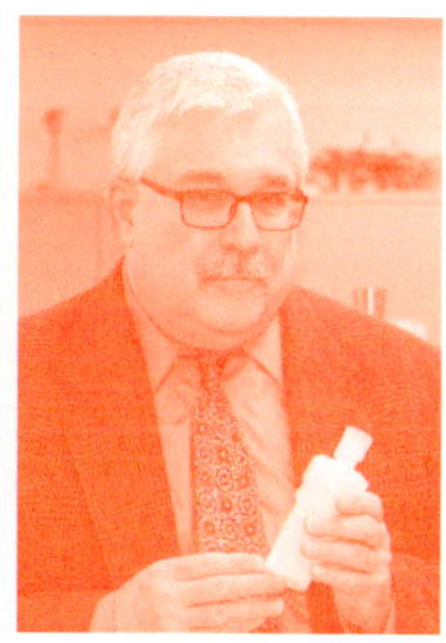
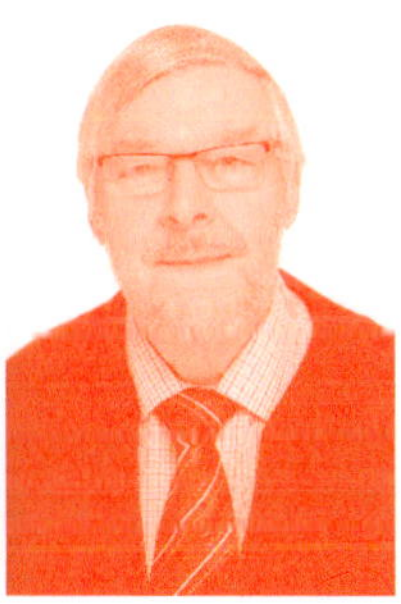
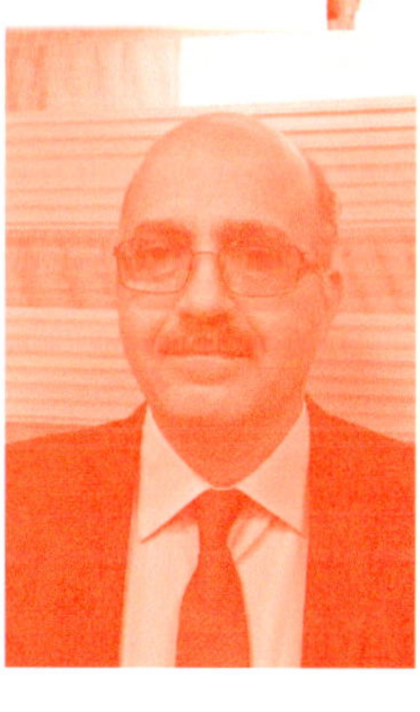
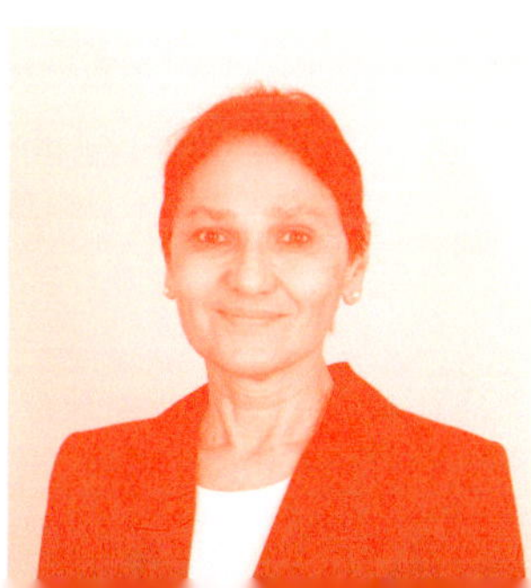
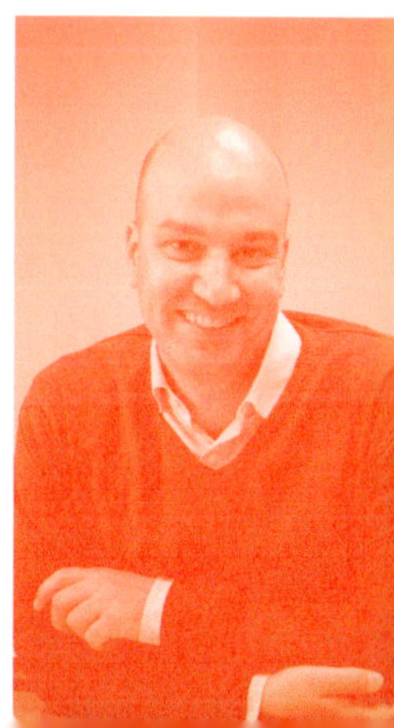

Hip Surgeries
http://dx.doi.org/10.5772/intechopen.80059
Edited by Nahum Rosenberg

Contributors
Gerard Sheridan, James Cashman, Fiona Dobson, Michelle Hall, Laura Diamond, Kim Allison, Carlos Roberto Galia, Fernando Pagnussato, Tiango Aguiar Ribeiro, Cristiano Valter Diesel, Marcelo Reuwsaat Guimarães, Yavuz Selim Kabukçuoğlu, Yaşar Mahsut Dinçel, Mehmet Ümit Çetin, Nahum Rosenberg

First published in London, United Kingdom, 2019 by IntechOpen
IntechOpen is the global imprint of INTECHOPEN LIMITED, registered in England and Wales, registration number: 11086078, The Shard, 25th floor, 32 London Bridge Street
London, SE19SG – United Kingdom
Printed in Croatia

British Library Cataloguing-in-Publication Data
A catalogue record for this book is available from the British Library

Additional hard copies can be obtained from orders@intechopen.com

Hip Surgeries
Edited by Nahum Rosenberg
p. cm.
Print ISBN 978-1-83880-235-6
Online ISBN 978-1-83880-236-3

For EU product safety concerns:
IN TECH d.o.o., Prolaz Marije Krucifikse Kozulić 3, 51000 Rijeka, Croatia,
info@intechopen.com or visit our website at intechopen.com.

Meet the editor

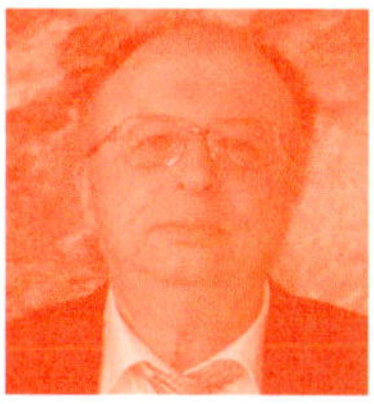

Rosenberg Nahum, MD, MOrth (Hons), FRCS (England), is an orthopedic surgeon holding an MD degree from Technion-ITT, which he received in 1990. He did a residency in orthopedic surgery at Rambam Medical Center, Haifa, between 1990 and 1997. He received his MOrth, Nuffield Fellow (Orthopedic Surgery), from Oxford University in 1998/99, and his Fellowship in Orthopedic Surgery at the University of Nottingham in 2002. He has been a senior orthopedic surgeon at Rambam Health Care Campus since 2003 and an assistant clinical professor in the Faculty of Medicine, Technion-ITT, Haifa, since 2007. He is a member of the editorial boards of eight scientific journals. His research interests include the outcome of orthopedic procedures and bone biology.

Contents

Preface

Hip surgery is one of the most challenging branches in orthopedic surgery because of the ultimate role of the hip joint in weight bearing during movement. Its role is especially crucial because of the limited ability of external orthotic devices to bear weight when the hip is disarranged, unstable, and painful. Therefore, orthopedic surgery advancement started with hip surgery, and from the experience gained with this joint, surgical methods for the treatment other large joints have evolved.

In this book the authors attempt to present the current knowledge on hip surgery methods in relation to joint anatomy, biomechanics, and the design of the surgical solution. Accordingly, data on the anticipated outcomes from different hip surgeries is described. The book focuses special attention on surgical decision making in hip surgery according to the treated pathology.

Dr. Nahum Rosenberg
Department of Traumatology,
Orthopedics and Disaster Surgery,
I.M. Sechenov First Moscow State Medical University,
Moscow, Russia

Orthopedics Department,
Rambam Health Care Campus,
Haifa, Israel

Chapter 1

Introductory Chapter: Hip Surgeries

Nahum Rosenberg

1. Introduction

> *"The present progress in surgery is so rapid that one year now is like a former hundred, and ten can leave us not outstripped but at the post."* Arnold H. Henry [1].

Hip surgery intends to treat disabling conditions in hip joint that cannot be resolved by conservative means, either by pharmacological or by mechanical aids. Without proper therapeutically solution, the individual with hip disability will lose the capability of independency that relies of unsupported and independent ambulation. Naturally this fact is a driven force for the development and improvement of surgical techniques and implants in hip surgeries.

Generally, surgical solutions are required as acute solutions in hip trauma and as salvage procedure in chronic hip arthritis. As expected, sometimes the surgical solutions for either can be utilized for both; e.g., endoprosthesis implantations are used for treatment of femoral neck fractures although initially developed for arthritic conditions, and internal fixation hardware is used for femoral and pelvic osteotomies to improve hip biomechanics in developmental hip abnormalities although the internal fixation concept was mainly designed for fracture treatment.

Hip joint has a sophisticated mechanical design that allows body weight-bearing and lower limb movement but the initial attempts to solve its malfunction by the mechanical means only obviously failed. When the biological aspects were not addressed sufficiently, the implants' characteristics alone were not enough for the long-term weight-bearing and hip joint stability. As such, the Smith-Petersen nail for the proximal femur fixation had to be evolved eventually to the compression concepts of sliding nails to enable compression of the fracture and reduce stresses on the metallic nail that usually cause either the brakeage of the nail or its cutting through the bone. Similarly, the initial "mechanistic" attempts in the hip arthroplasty by Themistokles Gluck, Philip Wiles, Marius Smith Petersen, and others in the nineteenth century, who tried to replace the damaged hip joint by artificial implant, failed because of the insufficient material properties of the implants during the joint friction with subsequential implant loosening [2]. The recognition of the crucial importance of the biocompatibility and stress bearing properties by the implant components gave the breakthrough by Sir John Charnley whose implant reached survivorship of more than 20 years postoperatively, e.g., 78% 35 years survivorship [3]. These issues are discussed in this book with additional emphasis on surgical techniques and approaches that also evolved gradually aiming to reduce or eliminate the rate of implants failure, dislocations, and loosening, septic and aseptic.

It should be emphasized that the rapid development of new techniques and implants in hip surgery, besides bringing a desired relieve for patients, can possess unexpected failures that have not been foreseen during the initial design. Therefore, an extra caution should be exercised during implementation of new techniques and

IntechOpen

technologies. Statistical survivorship evaluation, especially for the new implants, by a specially designed survivorship analysis [4, 5] can reduce the danger of the widespread use of failing designs.

The authors of the chapters of the book described extensively the various techniques and surgical approaches which are currently practiced in hip surgery. They provide a review for young surgeons who aim to join this exciting field of orthopedic surgery, and the experienced surgeons probably will enjoy the knowledge sharing and aspirational ideas of the authors.

Author details

Nahum Rosenberg

1 Department of Traumatology, Orthopedics and Disaster Surgery, I.M. Sechenov First Moscow State Medical University, Moscow, Russia

2 Orthopedics Department, Rambam Health Care Campus, Haifa, Israel

*Address all correspondence to: nahumrosenberg@hotmail.com

References

[1] Henry AK. Extensile Exposure. Third Edition. Churchill Livinston 1995, pp.viii

[2] Ellis H. The Cambridge Illustrated History of Surgery. Cambridge University Press, UK 2009. pp. 164

[3] Callaghan JJ et al. Survivorship of a Charnley total hip arthroplasty. A concise follow-up, at a minimum of thirty-five years, of previous reports. Journal of Bone and Joint Surgery. American Volume. 2009 Nov;**91**(11):2617-2621. DOI: 10.2106/JBJS.H.01201

[4] Rosenberg N, Soudry M. Survivorship analysis of orthopedic procedures – Practical approach. Arthroscopy. 2011;**27**(Suppl 4):16-24

[5] Murray DW, Carr AJ, Bulstrode C. Survival Analysis of Joint Replacements. Journal of Bone and Joint Surgery [Br]. 1993; 75-B: 697-704

Chapter 2

Osteoarthritis of the Hip Joint

Gerard A. Sheridan and James P. Cashman

Abstract

The incidence of osteoarthritis of the hip is increasing internationally. With the population becoming older and the rates of obesity increasing on a global scale, we are seeing more traumatic and idiopathic degeneration of the native hip joint. The pathological processes occurring in the hip have been described at a macroscopic and microscopic level. The inability of surface hyaline cartilage to heal is one of the major contributors to the irreversible nature of degeneration once it begins. Many classification systems have been described to characterise the extent of disease. History and examination play a pivotal role in the management algorithm. The goals of treatment are to improve pain, function and quality of life. Numerous non-operative treatments exist as do many operative interventions. Total hip arthroplasty is arguably the most successful operation developed in orthopaedic surgery to date. We discuss the condition of osteoarthritis as it pertains to the hip and we consider the patients' course from onset of symptoms through their investigation up to their definitive management.

Keywords: hip, osteoarthritis, osteotomy, total hip arthroplasty, revision total hip arthroplasty

1. Introduction

The hip joint is a ball and socket-type joint which is commonly affected by degenerative changes leading to osteoarthritis. Osteoarthritis of the hip is a non-inflammatory arthrosis caused by progressive loss of cartilage on the surface of the femoral head and the acetabulum. These two surfaces articulate normally with smooth lubricated motion. This allows painless weight-bearing through the normal hip joint and efficient mobilisation. When cartilaginous changes take place on the joint surface, degeneration occurs. This in turn leads to pain, restricted range of motion and limited function for those affected by the condition. These are the main clinical hallmarks found in osteoarthritis of the hip.

In the United States of America, the incidence of osteoarthritis is reported as 8 per 100,000 patients. Osteoarthritis of the hip is the main surgical indication for total hip arthroplasty [1]. Studies from the UK have demonstrated that osteoarthritis has an incidence of 9 in 1000 at-risk adults every year [2]. Yu et al. state that these figures are consistent across the international community. It is reasonable to take these figures as representative of the incidence of osteoarthritis in the developed world. Developing countries may demonstrate different incidences of osteoarthritis however. Unfortunately, robust data is not easily available for all countries in this area.

2. Aetiology

There are two commonly accepted aetiologies for osteoarthritis of the hip. These fall loosely under the headings of genetic causes and environmental causes.

2.1 Genetics

The genetic elements contributing to the condition have not yet been fully characterised. Pollard et al. assessed the risk of developing hip osteoarthritis in a population with a genetic predisposition. It was found that even when controlling for confounding variables, having a relative with hip osteoarthritis was associated with a significantly higher risk of developing the condition when compared to a population without any genetic predisposition [3]. Identification of a causative gene has yet to be confirmed. Defects in the *Col2 gene* (which codes for typ. 2 collagen, the main collagen type found in articular cartilage) may play a role in the development of hip osteoarthritis from a genetic perspective [4]. In 2015, Prof. A.J. Carr of Oxford was the senior author on the work entitled 'Osteoarthritis' which was published in The Lancet journal that year. The group references the arcOGEN consortium which had identified 11 genetic loci at the time associated with Osteoarthritis [5]. Carr also references the role of single nucleotide polymorphisms and how they may explain the genetic role in osteoarthritis by coding for BMI, bone mineral density and hip morphologies in the affected populations [5]. One can appreciate the significant role that genetics seems to play in this condition.

2.2 Environment

Environmental factors contributing to osteoarthritis of the hip are much better understood. The hip joint is a mechanical entity that relies on a number of key concepts for its functioning.

2.2.1 Lubrication

There are many types of lubrication described which will be discussed in detail later in this chapter. The hip is a synovial joint and fluid-film lubrication predominates in this type of joint [6]. The main purpose of lubrication is to reduce friction between two opposing surfaces in motion. Friction is described by the ***following equation [6]:

$$F = \mu_f \times W$$

In this equation, F = frictional force, μ_f is the coefficient of friction for a given material and W is the applied load. It follows that the lower the coefficient of friction for a surface bearing is, the less frictional load and wear that surface will undergo. When lubrication of a joint is insufficient to prevent friction, wear and degeneration occur. This is the mechanism by which obesity and heavy manual labour contribute to osteoarthritis in the hip.

2.2.2 Congruency

A congruent joint is one that has a uniform surface in contact with another uniform surface. Wear is defined as the progressive loss of a bearing substance (i.e. cartilage) as a result of chemical or mechanical action [6]. In the case of an incongruent joint, mechanical wear occurs at a much higher rate because the loss of uniform surfaces in contact means that focal stresses are much higher and lubrication is much less effective. An example of this would be a femoral head fracture. This is a rare traumatic injury but rates of post-traumatic arthritis have been reported as high as 20% [7]. Acetabular fractures have been known to lead to contribute to post-traumatic arthritis of the hip. Magala et al. described the importance of joint congruency as it relates to the hip. It was found that patients with undisplaced fractures of the acetabulum had significantly better functional outcomes then those who sustained a displaced fracture of the acetabulum. This illustrates the importance of joint surface congruity, and how disturbance of this can lead to accelerated degeneration and poor functional performance of the hip joint [8]. Paediatric conditions such as Perthes disease, regular use of steroids and fractures to the neck of femur may all eventually result in avascular necrosis of the femoral head causing incongruity of the joint with resulting osteoarthritis of the hip as described. Avascular necrosis is the process of cell death secondary to vascular insufficiency. Bones with tenuous blood supplies are more predisposed to developing this condition. Any bone can sustain this injury but the commonest bones with a classically poor blood supply include the scaphoid, the talus and of course the femoral head. Subchondral bone loses its integrity leading to collapse, articular incongruity and rapid degenerative changes in the joint leading to significant functional limitations and pain in many cases.

2.2.3 Contact surface area

The hip joint is composed of a spherical head that rotates within a socket (acetabulum). The acetabulum covers the femoral head superiorly allowing forces to be transmitted up from the lower limbs to the pelvis and up through the spine during gait. The amount of force being transmitted depends on the mass of the body and the surface area of the hip joint.

'Stress' is defined as the 'force per unit area applied' and it is measured in N/m^2 [6]. For a given force (body mass) acting across the hip joint, the stress level at the joint surface will vary depending on the amount of acetabular and femoral head surface in contact. When the acetabulum covers a large amount of the femoral head, two large surface areas are in contact. This leads to lower contact stresses at the joint surface

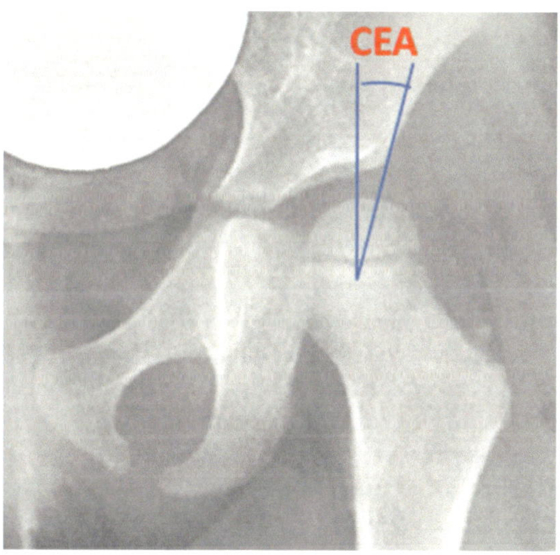

Figure 1.
Centre-edge angle demonstrated on a paediatric pelvis.

with reduced wear and enhanced joint preservation. When the acetabular surface area is small (e.g. in developmental dysplasia of the hip), the contact stresses across the hip joint are very high leading to accelerated degeneration and wear rates. In developmental dysplasia of the hip (DDH), the hip joint does not form normally. This leads to a spectrum of disease from poor femoral head coverage to dislocation in utero. The centre-edge angle (CEA) is a measurement used to quantify the amount of coverage provided to the femoral head by the acetabulum. Hips with larger CEAs have higher surface areas in contact leading to less wear and degeneration. Terjesen looked at the effect of CEA on the development of hip osteoarthritis in a population with DDH. It was found that patients with a normal CEA (20° or above) had only a 5% risk of developing hip osteoarthritis. Patients with an abnormal CEA (<20°) had a 22% chance of developing hip osteoarthritis. This demonstrates the significance of the contact surface area in the native hip and its role in the aetiology of hip degeneration (**Figure 1**).

3. Pathology

3.1 Cartilage constituents

Before describing the pathological processes that occur in the process or osteoarthritis we will first consider the normal constitution of articular cartilage. As with most connective tissues, articular cartilage consists of cells (chondrocytes) contained within an extracellular matrix. This extracellular matrix contains many elements as described by Ramachandran [6]:

- Fibres (collagen, elastin)
- Water (75% of wet weight)
- Proteoglycans
- Glycosaminoglycans
- Glycoproteins
- Matrix metalloproteinases
- Extracellular ions

The two major matrix components are the collagen fibres and the proteoglycans. Collagen mostly present in cartilage is type II. Three α-chains are arranged in a triple helix formation. This forms a collagen molecule which is then arranged in a quarter-staggered array. Collagen is essential for the integrity of the extracellular matrix of cartilage. Proteoglycans are molecules consisting of glycosaminoglycans (GAGs). Glycosaminoglycans such as keratan-sulphate and chondroitin-sulphate have a negative charge. This negative charge attracts cations and water which contributes to the osmotic pressure within cartilage and therefore the compressive strength of cartilage aggrecan is bound by a sugar bond to a hyaluronic acid backbone to form the proteoglycan aggregate. These proteoglycan aggregates entwine with collagen fibres and chondrocytes to form the majority of the microstructure of articular cartilage [6].

Glycoproteins are macromolecules such as laminin and lubricin that are dispersed throughout the synovial fluid to act as a lubricant for the articulating joint surface. The role of lubricin was investigated by Galicia et al. [9]. It was postulated that pro-inflammatory markers were increased in an osteoarthritis population requiring total joint arthroplasty. When the arthroplasty group were compared to a control group, it was found that levels of IL-6, IL-8, VEGF, IL-1β, MCP-1, EGF, and TNF-α were significantly increased [9]. These proinflammatory markers were raised in the arthroplasty group both preoperatively and postoperatively. Of note, compared to the controls, lubricin levels were decreased. The implication of these findings is that a traumatic event may induce a cascade of increased pro-inflammatory markers in osteoarthritic patients. This cascade seems to reduce the levels of lubricin circulating in the synovial fluid of the joint. This may explain one of the mechanisms responsible for post-traumatic arthritis development.

There are various enzymes present in the hip joint which can either destroy or preserve cartilage. Once these enzymes are balanced with a certain homeostasis, normal cartilage integrity will be preserved. If however the destructive enzymes are more prominent than the protective enzymes, there will be a nett loss of cartilage tissue. There are two main enzymes responsible for cartilage degradation: aggrecanase and collagenase [4]. These two enzymes are known as matrix metalloproteinases (MMPs). Other MMPs include gelatinases, stromelysins, matrilysins and membrane-type MMPs [10]. Aggrecanase is responsible for the degradation of proteoglycans (e.g. aggrecan), an example being ADAMT. Another type of MMP is collagenase. Collagenase degrades collagen found in the substance of the articular cartilage of the hip. An example of this MMP would be MMP-13. IL-1β is a substance found in the synovium which has a role in the activation of MMPs. It also activates nuclear factor κβ (NF-κβ). IF it were possible to reduce the activation of these MMPs by inhibiting IL-1β, the downstream effect would be cartilaginous preservation in the hip joint. A study published in February 2018 by Zhang et al. investigated this effect [11]. This study was analysing the in vitro effect of isoliquiritigenin on primary cultured chondrocytes. By analysing mRNA and protein expression levels, inhibition of MMP expression by isoliquiritigenin was assessed. In vitro studies were also performed on mice articular cartilage. Final results confirmed a reduction in the expression of MMPs and a reduced activation of NF-κβ. They concluded that this pathway may be targeted in future to treat osteoarthritis of articular joints.

There are two enzymes responsible for inhibition of the MMPs. These are known as tissue inhibitors of matrix metalloproteinases (TIMPs) and plasminogen activator inhibitor-1 (PAI-1). The ratio of MMP to TIMP has a role in determining the nett MMP activity, ECM turnover and tissue remodelling [10]. This is an antibiotic traditionally used to treat infections such as chlamydia. This has a broad systemic mechanism of action and therefore as many unwanted side effects. Liu et al. report that newer, highly targeted TIMP therapy may reduce the generic musculoskeletal side effects traditionally associated with TIMP therapy which may allow a more widespread uptake of the medication to treat osteoarthritis in the population [10].

3.2 Cartilage structure

Articular cartilage is arranged in a series of layers which all play a role in the diverse functions of the cartilage at different levels. The most superficial layer is the lamina splendens which contains long collagen fibres (mainly type II collagen) orientated parallel to the joint surface. This layer has flat chondrocytes, high concentrations of water and low concentrations of proteoglycans. This layer also has the greatest tensile stiffness [4]. Collagen fibres and chondrocytes are oriented parallel to the surface to resist shear forces. Shear is the type of force generated when two opposing surfaces in contact move in opposite directions.

Longitudinal fibres at a perpendicular orientation to the joint surface would be poorly adapted to cope with shear stresses on the surface cartilage. As the depth of the articular cartilage increases, fibres and cells are oriented in a diagonal fashion. This essentially acts as a 'transition zone' to allow smooth progression from the superficial lamina splendens described above and the deeper layers of articular cartilage. In the deep radial zone, fibres are aligned to withstand compressive forces. This deep layer has a low water content and high proteoglycan content compared to the more superficial layers. Fibres and cells run perpendicular to the joint surface. This gives a mechanical advantage to the deep cartilage in compression. The arrangement of deep fibres in the radial zone allows the cartilage to withstand this compression.

Deep to the radial layer is the tidemark. The tidemark is composed of type X collagen. It demarcates the boundary between the flexible superficial cartilage and the deep calcified cartilage in the calcified zone [4]. Deep to the tidemark is the calcified zone of cartilage which then blends with subchondral bone completing the transition between cartilage superficially to bone in the deep layers.

Understanding the structure of cartilage is imperative to understanding how and why osteoarthritis develops the way it does. The lamina splendens as described is essential for the frictionless motion of one joint surface in contact with another. With loss of this layer, surface irregularities begin to manifest and loading across the joint surface becomes less uniform leading to focal areas of high loading with increased wear rates for the joint overall. Ramachandran describes the process of structural change in cartilage with the progression of osteoarthritis [6]. Firstly, collagen is disrupted, either through direct trauma or else via the MMP mechanism already described. Interference of this meshwork then allows proteoglycans to attract more water. This has an effect on the 'Young's modulus of elasticity' of the articular cartilage. This modulus (depicted by the symbol 'ε') is a measure of the materials behaviour when a certain level of stress (or load) is applied to that material. For materials with a high Young's modulus, a high level of stress will cause a relatively low amount of strain (material displacement/movement) compared to materials with a lower modulus. This applies to the hip joint in the following way: with osteoarthritis, collagen is degraded, and water content increases due to more proteoglycan exposure. This increased amount of water lowers the Young's modulus meaning that when a load is placed through the joint, a higher level of strain or displacement will occur in the substance of the cartilage. Essentially the cartilage is now less stiff and so is more likely to deform and become damaged through the normal weight-bearing process. In this way, the macroscopic degeneration of cartilage is a synergistic process of degradation where one flaw in structural integrity increases the likelihood of developing a further flaw in the structure.

Based on the above discussion, Ramachandran proposes three main reasons for the observed effect of cartilage deformation [6]:

1. Collagen-proteoglycan matrix disruption
2. Large interstitial fluid movements causing loss of proteoglycan and decreased stiffness
3. Rapid repeated high loading leaving no time for stress relaxation and repair of collagen-proteoglycan matrix

Again, the key to understanding this vast limitation in this tissue can be found in the structure of the tissue. The layered configuration of cartilage has many implications in relation to its healing. In 1980, a classic study published by Mitchell et al. observed the essential role of the tidemark in cartilage healing. Using micron electroscopy and various staining techniques in rabbit models, they found that cartilaginous defects tended to heal due to the proliferation of a cell population emanating from the tide mark [12]. The tide mark marks the boundary between flexible superficial cartilage and deep stiff calcified cartilage. In 1993, Shapiro et al. described the morphological composition of tissue that fills the void of cartilaginous defects in full-thickness defects of articular cartilage [13]. Defects were made in the cartilage of New-Zealand white rabbits down to the tidemark. It was found that the tissue type to replace the deficient area was a type of cartilage known as fibrocartilage. If the cartilage sustains an injury more superficial than the tide mark, the defect will simply remain without any healing or regeneration. This is due in part to the relatively avascular nature of this part of the tissue. If then the femoral head of the hip were to sustain an injury of its cartilage that were deep enough to violate the tidemark, Shapiro has shown that regenerative tissue will form. It is very important to note however that this 'new cartilage' is fibrocartilage and not hyaline cartilage. Fibrocartilage has some differing features when compared with to hyaline cartilage. This consists mostly of typ. 1 collagen, unlike hyaline cartilage which consists of typ. 2 collagen. Importantly, fibrocartilage is not designed for weight bearing like hyaline cartilage is since it has a higher coefficient of friction when compared to hyaline cartilage. In this way, articular cartilage does have the capacity to regenerate and heal defects that fulfil a certain set of criteria. This regeneration however is not optimal for the function intended in articular joints, and so once the articular cartilage is injured, it is fair to say that it will never be normal again.

In the 1970s, Maroudas and Venn published their work describing the physiology of cartilage as we know it today. The classic picture of increased water content and reduced glycosaminoglycans was detailed in this seminal work [14].

4. History

When considering the symptoms associated with osteoarthritis of the hip, pain and function are the two biggest contributors to the natural history. A precise description of the pain is essential to obtain in the history. Usually, patients will describe an aching type of pain in the groin. There may be contributing areas such as the greater trochanter and buttock but the groin for the most part is the site of complaint. This pain usually has an insidious onset. The traditional description of osteoarthritic pain is one that is less severe in the morning and with rest. The traditional teaching is that exercise and progression through the day towards evening time will be associated with deterioration of pain and symptoms throughout the day. It is well established that significant weight gain may be associated with significant deterioration in the patients reported symptoms. In early stages of osteoarthritis, reversal of this effect through weight loss can be seen in a number for cases. The reason for this association is simply related to the load passing through the hip joint, as the overall body mass increases, the force per unit area (N/m^2) or 'stress' passing through the hip joint is significantly increased. Subjective pain is also significantly affected by the patients' general psychological status. It is well described that patients suffering from depression and other disorders are poorly adapted to cope with pain and may experience subjectively higher levels of pain when compared to a patient that does not have depression but does have the same level of osteoarthritis on radiographic examination.

It is important to consider a number of factors in relation to pain. In 1891, in his series of lectures relating to "rest and pain", Hilton described a very important fundamental principle in orthopaedics [15]. Hiltons' law states that "the nerve supplying a joint also supplies the muscles that traverse the joint and the skin sensation over that joint". It follows that when a nerve traverses more than one joint, pain actually originating in the knee for example may manifest as pain in the hip and vice versa. In this way, hip osteoarthritis may actually present as pain in the knee or the lumbar spine. Therefore, a good rule of thumb in orthopaedic practice is to always examine the joint above and below the area of complaint.

The effect of pain on the patient's life is essential to characterise. If the pain is deteriorating, it is important to confirm over what time frame and whether there are is any specific exacerbating activity. Often, avoidance of the activity leading to the pain is enough to reduce symptoms to a level acceptable to the patient. In this way, lifestyle modification and activity limitation can play a role in the early conservative management of early osteoarthritis. It is important for patients to stay active however. Muscle deconditioning around the hip and weight gain in general are associated with poorer hip function and deterioration in the symptom profile of the patient. Jeanmaire et al. described the effect of low lean mass on the quality of life and function of patients with osteoarthritis of the hip [16]. They concluded that having less lean mass (i.e. a deconditioned hip with poor strength) is associated with poorer quality of life and poorer function in this cohort. This emphasises the importance of strengthening exercises and remaining active in this cohort. This can be a very difficult cohort of patients to treat, especially because of the known association with high BMI rates and infection of implanted total hip replacements. At a mean follow-up of 3 years, Pulos et al. described a higher rate of total hip replacement revision for infection. This was seen if the patients BMI was over 35 [17]. This illustrates the complex relationship between pain profiles, patient BMI and surgical infection as experienced by many orthopaedic hip surgeons.

Other factors to consider in the history are past medical and past surgical history. Rondon et al. assessed the complications of performing total hip and knee replacements in patients with Parkinson's disease. It was shown that the risk of periprosthetic fracture and dislocation were significantly higher in this patient cohort when compared to patients without Parkinson's disease [18]. In the patient with neurological dysfunction, proprioceptive awareness and motor control are commonly lacking. In the initial postoperative phase, stringent limitations are placed on the patient regarding acceptable positions of the hip to prevent the risk of dislocation in both the acute and chronic settings. If the patient is unable to adhere to these instructions, they are at much higher risk of dislocation and chronic instability. Instability episodes may also lead to falls and fractures which are very significant injuries in this frail cohort of patient.

5. Examination

Examination is an essential part in the management algorithm of patients with hip osteoarthritis. Patients should be examined under the following headings.

5.1 Inspection

Much information can be ascertained through inspection alone. Scars, swellings, muscle wasting (particularly in the gluteal and quadriceps region), asymmetry and deformity are essential to comment on in the examination of the hip.

Sagittal alignment should reveal the presence of any fixed flexion deformity in the hip. Patients will often compensate for this malalignment by flexing the knee and plantarflexing the ankle to maintain foot contact with the floor. A hyperlordosis of the lumbar spine may mask the severity of a fixed flexion contracture. This can be objectively evaluated using Thomas' test. This will be discussed in turn.

5.2 Gait

Gait analysis will often show an antalgic gait. This is when the patient demonstrates a shortened stance phase on the side of the affected hip due to pain on weight bearing. Other abnormal patterns of gait include Trendelenburg gait. This occurs due to weakness or painful inhibition of the hip abductors during gait. During single leg stance on the affected side, the planted foot acts as a fixed support for the body. To clear the contralateral leg during its swing phase, the abductors contract thereby lifting the contralateral pelvis and allowing foot clearance.

Another type of gait that occurs is the fused hip gait. Typically, these patients have no terminal stance and they may present with an exaggerated lumbar lordosis also.

Limb length discrepancy manifests either through circumduction of the long leg, ankle plantarflexion of the short leg or hip vaulting of the long leg through hip flexion. Patients may become very good at compensating for a leg length discrepancy, so the clinical suspicion should be high for his abnormality in the preoperative setting. Coleman blocks should be used to evaluate the degree of clinical discrepancy as perceived by the patient.

5.3 Limb length discrepancy (LLD)

It has frequently been described after total hip replacement that limb length discrepancy remains a very significant complication. It has often been quoted as the main reason for patient dissatisfaction and is also noted to be the commonest reason for litigation against orthopaedic surgeons in the postoperative period [19]. For this reason, it is imperative to identify the presence of any preoperative limb length discrepancy. This can be allowed for in the surgical technique utilised by the surgeon. Regardless of the surgical technique, the most important point is to notice it in the preoperative setting.

There are many ways of assessing the clinical limb length discrepancy. The use of Coleman blocks has already been described and these are very useful tools to have available in the out-patient setting. Firstly, the true and apparent limb lengths should be attained. The true limb length is measured as the distance from the anterior superior iliac spine (ASIS) on the pelvis down to the medial malleolus. The apparent limb length discrepancy includes the adaptive mechanisms that the patient has developed and gives an indication to the LLD that the patient feels subjectively. The apparent LLD does not give a measure of the true length discrepancy in the lower limbs. If it is confirmed that there is indeed a true LLD, the next step is to characterise where exactly in the lower limb this is coming from: the tibia, the femur or the hip.

The Galeazzi test is used to identify where the discrepancy may be originating from. To perform the test, the patient is laid supine, hips are flexed to 45° and the knees are flexed to 90°. The ankles are brought together at the level of the medial malleoli and the knees are then observed. On lateral inspection, if the right patella is lower and more distal to the left, it is likely that the shortening is coming from the right tibia. If the right patella is lower and more proximal to the left, it is likely that the right femur is shorter than the left. If the femur is the suspected source of shortening, one must proceed to perform the digital Bryant's test. Again, the patient is still supine. A line is drawn directly vertical down from both ASIS's. The tip of the GT is palpated bilaterally, and a line is drawn perpendicular to the line drawn from the ASIS. This horizontal line passes from the tip of the GT on both sides and ends once it intersects with the vertical line passing vertically down from the ASIS. If there is a discrepancy in the length of these two lines, one can assume that the source of femoral shortening is supratrochanteric. If these two lines are equal bilaterally, one can assume that the source of femoral shortening is below the level of the trochanters.

5.4 Palpation and motion

Finally, then, one should ask the patient to identify the source of pain. Classically the patient will point to the groin region. Assure the patient that you will try to avoid causing them pain during the examination, but this is not always possible. Begin palpating away from the source of pain initially and then migrate towards the site of pain then.

After joint palpation, motion should then be assessed. Firstly, the presence of contractures should be documented. Thomas' test has been described to eliminate any compensatory lumbar lordosis developed by the patient [20]. In a patient with a fixed flexion deformity (FFD) of the hip, hyperlordosis of the lumbar spine often occurs to improve the overall hip extension and to allow improved gait patterns. To perform the test, place your flattened hand behind the patient's lumbar spine and ask them to flatten their back. This eliminated the lumbar curvature. Then place your other hand behind the patient's ipsilateral knee, ask them to extend the knee and compress the popliteal fossa against your hand. Patients with an FFD will be unable to perform this and the angle subtended by the bed and the posterior aspect of the flexed femur is the fixed flexion angle of the hip joint.

Before assessing active and passive ranges of motion in the hip joint, the hip must be squared to expose any coronal contractures of the hips and allow a more accurate comparison of the ranges in both hips. Firstly, ask the patient to show their active range of motion (ROM). An initial straight leg raise will show the strength of the hip and potentially reveal a contributing spinal aetiology to the pain if Lasègue's test is positive. Document the hip flexion, abduction and adduction with the pelvis squared. With the hip and knee flexed to 90°, document the range of internal and external rotation of the hip. A very common finding is impingement indicated by pain at the ends of the rotational range of motion. Stinchfield's test may be performed. The hip is flexed to 30° with the knee in extension. The patient is asked to flex the femur up against resistance. Pain induced by this examination implies an intraarticular source to the pain.

Place the patient in the lateral position then and assess abductor strength. Hip extension is also easily assessed in this position. Ober's test is used to identify ITB tightness as described above. To perform Ober's test, position the patient laterally and flex the lower hip to eliminate the lumbar lordosis. Then flex the upper knee to 90° while abducting and extending the hip. In patients with a tight ITB, the hip will remain passively abducted and will not adduct as the lateral structures of the thigh are either too painful or too tight to allow passive adduction [20]. Piriformis test can be performed in this position by flexing the knee to 90° and the hip to 60°. Downward pressure on the painful leg reproduces pain.

Next, place the patient prone. Assess gluteal bulk and hip extension again in this position. The lumbar spine and sacroiliac joints are easily palpated in this position. Prone is the best position to assess the version of the femur. Craig's test is used to assess the proximal femur version [20]. Flex the knee to 90° and hold the ankle in one hand. Internally and externally rotate the hip joint whilst palpating the greater trochanter (GT). When the trochanter feels most prominent, this is when the femoral neck is parallel to the floor. If the GT is most prominent with 15° of internal rotation of the hip, his means that the femoral neck has an anteversion angle of about 15°. If the GT is most prominent in 23° of external rotation of the hip, this means that the femoral neck is 23° retroverted.

Finally, one must never forget to examine the knee and lumbar spine when performing the hip examination.

6. Investigations

6.1 Radiography

Investigations used in hip osteoarthritis are dominated by the simple plain radiograph. An adequate X-ray of the pelvis will allow characterisation of the disease extent and even detailed preoperative planning in the vast majority of cases. There are 4 radiographic findings classically described when describing osteoarthritis of the hip joint:

1. Loss of joint space

2. Osteophyte formation

3. Subchondral sclerosis

4. Subchondral cysts

This can be represented simply by the mnemonic 'LOSS'. Loss of cartilage through the pathological mechanisms already discussed leads to an approximation of the acetabular and femoral bone on plain radiograph. With disease progression, the bony ends appear to be in direct contact due to the complete destruction of all articular cartilage. Cartilage is not ossified in the normal hip and so it is radiolucent giving the appearance of an apparent 'joint space'. Loss of cartilage therefore gives rise to a loss of this joint space.

Osteophytes are the metaplastic osseous and cartilaginous tissues found at the rim of articular surfaces of joints that experience subtle instability. The may play a number of roles including protection of articular cartilage and redistribution stresses borne by the hip joint [21]. Interestingly, Tsurumoto et al. described the relationship between the severity of stress experienced by an osteoarthritic joint and the size of osteophyte. It was demonstrated that joints subjected to higher stresses were likely to develop larger osteophytes [22]. In this way, osteophytes may act as a surrogate marker for the severity of degeneration in the hip. Due to microscopic and macroscopic changes in the structural integrity of cartilage, areas of weakening develop. These are known as subchondral cysts. Areas of reactive sclerosis develop as a generic response to injury. This accounts for the common radiographic finding of subchondral cysts and subchondral sclerosis observed in severe cases of hip osteoarthritis (**Figure 2**).

Many classification systems have been developed to try and create an accurate way of describing radiographic findings. There are numerous classifications used to describe osteoarthritis throughout the years. In 1963, Kellgren described 4 grades of osteoarthritis based on the progressive observation of osteophytes, sclerosis, joint space narrowing, femoral head deformity and cyst formation [23]. In 1990, Croft et al. also described a classification system based on the progressive appearance of

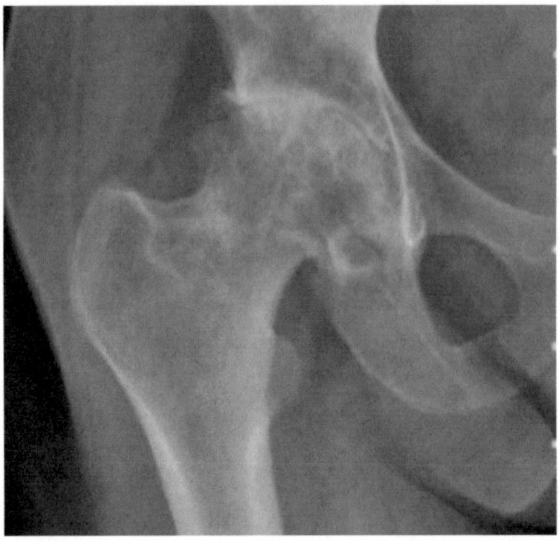

Figure 2.
Hip radiograph illustrating loss of joint space, femoral and acetabular osteophytes, femoral head subchondral sclerosis and acetabular subchondral cysts.

similar factors described by Kellgren. In 2005, Jacobsen et al. described a third classification system for osteoarthritis of the hip. This system was different to the proceeding two in that it included some level of accurate measurement. The Kellgren and Croft systems are clearly open to extensive inter-observer variability given the use of vague, non-specific terms to describe the stages of a condition. Jacobsen et al. looked at a specific measurement defined as the joint space width (JSW). Three measurements are taken between the weight-bearing surface of the femoral head and the surface of the acetabulum. If any of these three measurements are below 2 mm, this is defined as osteoarthritis. In 2012, Terjesen et al. performed an evaluation of the above three classification systems. They found that the JSW <2 mm system gave the highest rate of interobserver reliability. It was also the simplest system and so was felt to be the most useful classification system for assessment of osteoarthritis of the hip.

Magnetic resonance imaging (MRI) can play a role in the evaluation of osteoarthritis of the hip. It is mostly used to assess soft tissue pathology in and around the hip joint. There is more of a role for MRI in research. Delayed gadolinium-enhanced MRI of cartilage (dGEMRIC) can characterise the very subtle features of early osteoarthritis and so it is often used in the clinical research setting. Again, this is not a commonplace modality in the standard investigation of osteoarthritis.

7. Non-operative management

The aim of all treatment for osteoarthritis of the hip is to relieve pain and to improve function. Characterising and simplifying the patients presenting complaint will guide the decision and make it clear as to what management path to take. Red flags to be mindful of in the history include night time pain that wakes the patient from their sleep, progressively reducing walking distance due to pain and functional limitation to a level that is not acceptable to the patient. A very comprehensive examination will help to rule out contributing factors form sources besides the hip as described already. We will discuss the full spectrum of hip osteoarthritis management and outline the indications and concerns associated with each management path.

7.1 Non-pharmacological

Non-operative intervention is either pharmacological or non-pharmacological. Non-pharmacological methods include quadriceps strengthening, hip ROM exercises, manual therapy, gait assistance and gait aids. A walking stick will often help when held in the hand opposite to the symptomatic side of hip osteoarthritis. In terms of free-body diagrams, the stick reduces the moment of the body weight acting around the painful hip joint by providing a counter-moment in the opposite direction. The abductors need to work less, and the overall joint force reaction is reduced. Carrying a heavy item in the ipsilateral hand can have the same effect on the free-body diagram by assisting the abductor force and thereby reducing the work performed by the abductor mechanism.

Sharma recently analysed the effect of non-pharmacological and non-operative intervention in hip osteoarthritis [24]. It was found that pharmacological treatment for osteoarthritis is lacking and needs to be optimised as soon as possible in the clinical setting. With time to total hip replacement (THR) as the outcome measure, Svege et al. reported their findings of a long-term randomised trial. Patients were randomised either to education about their condition with appropriate non-operative interventions or education supplemented with exercise therapy. Exercise therapy and education were associated with a longer time to THR implying the beneficial role of exercise in treating this condition [25]. Anecdote would seem to suggest however that once a hip is significantly painful with degeneration confirmed on radiograph, then non-operative measures are unlikely to ever really succeed. Bennell et al. performed a well designed prospective double-blinded randomised control trial to assess the role for physical therapy in the management of hip osteoarthritis [26]. 102 patients with significantly painful osteoarthritis of the hip were included in the study. Forty-nine patients were in the active group. They underwent education, manual therapy, home exercise and gait aid as appropriate. The remaining 53 patients underwent a sham intervention consisting of a self-applied gel three times a week. The intervention lasted for 12 weeks in total and pain and functional scores were assessed for both groups. The use of physical therapy did not show any significant improvement in the pain and functional outcomes of that patient cohort. In conclusion, the non-pharmacological modalities are highly effective in treating osteoarthritis currently. Sharma mentions the need however, to reconcile acceptable physical activity levels with osteoarthritis progression in the future for better understanding of the condition.

7.2 Pharmacological

Pharmacological analgesic control of hip osteoarthritis is important as it often improves painful symptoms to a baseline that is tolerable to the patient thereby allowing them to function. This may achieve the two aims of management in hip osteoarthritis: namely pain control and restoration of function. The 'World Health Organisation' introduced a document entitled 'cancer pain relief' in 1986 [27]. This was a document aimed at introducing a graded system for the controlled introduction of opioids into a patient's analgesic regimen. This was specifically targeted at cancer patients originally but has been adapted as a good approach to managing pain in the majority of painful conditions. The ladder has three steps as follows (**Figure 3**):

Step 1		Non-opioid	Adjuvant
Step 2	Weak opioid	Non-opioid	Adjuvant
Step 3	Strong opioid	Non-opioid	Adjuvant

Figure 3.
WHO analgesic ladder.

Non-opioids consist of medications such as paracetamol and aspirin. These are drugs with low side effect profiles which is why they are the first step on the ladder. Once the non-opioid medications have been exhausted, adjuvant non-opioid medications should be added in step 1. COX-2 inhibitors include medications such as celecoxib. The advantage of selective COX-2 inhibition is the reduction in the unwanted gastric side effects. Gastric inhibition of COX results in reduced PGE_2 and PGI_2. Reduction of these prostaglandins in the stomach reduces blood flow, increases acid production and results in dyspepsia, nausea and gastritis [6]. With the use of agents like celecoxib, constant usage instead of intermittent usage has been associated with significantly less episodes of painful flares [28]. Celecoxib appears to be the commonest disease-modifying analgesic prescribed in this cohort with function primarily being through PG and cytokine levels in the joint [29]. Topical NSAIDs may have some role also. The British National Institute for Clinical Excellence (NICE guidelines) released in 2014, recommend the use of topical NSAIDS before the use of oral NSAIDs.

After the pain has exceeded the control of step 1. Step 2 in the ladder should be commenced. Step 2 sees the introduction of weak opioids such as codeine, dihydrocodeine and tramadol. Opioid analgesics act on mu (μ) receptors in the spinal cord and brain. Receptors are located mostly in the dorsal horn of the spinal cord and the thalamus. Strong opioids found on the third step of the ladder include the likes of morphine, fentanyl and oxycodone. Again, these agents have a more significant inhibitory effect on pain but the risk of side effects may outweigh treatment in many cases.

Once all oral options have been exhausted, intraarticular injections of corticosteroids should be considered. Most of the national and international guidelines available for hip osteoarthritis will recommend intraarticular steroid injection as a good option before surgery to temporise the operation and in some cases avoid operation. McCabe et al. reviewed five studies assessing the effect of intraarticular steroid injections for the hip [30]. They found a significant reduction in pain levels at 8 weeks post-injection. In 2017, Chambers et al. published their work assessing the effect of intraarticular steroid injections of the hip. The study included 456 patients in total. 106 patients received 2 or more injections and then underwent total hip replacement. A matched cohort of 350 patients received only 1 injection and then underwent total hip replacement. Postoperative prosthetic infection rates were reported in both groups. The 'single injection' group had a significantly lower infection rate at 2%. Those receiving 2 or more injections had an infection rate of 6.6% [31]. Perhaps a reasonable approach to this issue would be to offer multiple steroid injections to patients who will likely never have an operation-either due to comorbidity or volition. If one suspects that a patient will likely undergo a total hip replacement in the future, then it is reasonable to offer a single injection only and then consider operation.

8. Operative management

8.1 Non-arthroplasty techniques

We have discussed the role of hip pathology in the young adult and how both intraarticular and extraarticular deformities may contribute to early onset osteoarthritis of the hip. Hip arthroscopy is a practice that is becoming increasingly used to treat predisposing conditions for arthritis and indeed treat arthritic patients also. We know that the presence of labral tears leads to chondral damage and therefore the development of hip osteoarthritis [32]. Hip arthroscopy has a role in the treatment of labral tears, focal chondral lesions and even ligamentum teres tears. Byrd et al. described a beneficial role of arthroscopy in patients with the above findings in the setting of DDH and mechanical abnormality. Questions are often asked posed about the role hip arthroscopy plays in patients with established hip osteoarthritis. Kemp et al. performed a systematic review assessing 22 studies [33]. They looked at pain and functional improvements in patients undergoing hip arthroscopy. Patients were divided into two groups: those with osteoarthritis and those without. Findings suggested that hip arthroscopy does improve function and pain in patients with pre-existing osteoarthritis. Their improvement was not as marked as the non-degenerative patients. Predictors of conversion to THR included patient age and the severity of chondral damage.

Other non-arthroplasty techniques include proximal femoral and acetabular osteotomies. We will consider the commonest osteotomy used for the treatment of dysplasia in the young adult-the Bernese (or Ganz) periacetabular osteotomy. In 1988, Ganz described his original Bernese periacetabular osteotomy [34]. The goal of the surgery was to realign the acetabular orientation to improve joint congruency, increase joint surface contact area, reduce high focal stresses and ultimately preserve the hip joint in the young adult for as long as possible. The technique describes an anterior (Smith-Petersen) approach to the hip joint. Three cuts are made in the pelvis as follows: superior pubic ramus cut (complete), supraacetabular cut (complete and extraarticular), ischial cut (incomplete). Nine parameters were described by Clohisy et al. that should be checked in the operating room before finishing the operation [35]:

1. Surface (weight-bearing acetabulum) should be more horizontal with an inclination of 0–10°

2. Lateral femoral head coverage should be improved with an angle of 25 to 35°

3. Medial aspect of the femoral head should be within 5 to 10 mm of the ilioischial line (this may require medialisation of the femoral head depending on the position of the individual case)

4. Acetabular version should be correct (one can assess a retroverted acetabulum by observing the anterior and posterior acetabular wall lines. If retroversion has occurred, the classic "crossover sign" will be evident on imaging)

5. Anterior femoral head coverage should be improved to 20–25° on the false-profile view of the proximal femur (a false profile view of the femur is a lateral view with roughly 25° internal rotation of the whole body on that side. This will give a true lateral view of the femoral head as it is situated in the acetabulum. Only on this intraoperative view can the anterior femoral head coverage be commented on)

6. The correction produces a congruent joint

7. Adequate head–neck offset is present or has been produced with osteochondroplasty

8. Adequate internal fixation has been achieved with acceptable screw position

9. Hip flexion of at least 90° and hip abduction of at least 30° can be achieved on table before the end of the operation

This is a significant operation for the patient to undergo and it is not without complication. Patients undergoing PAO (periacetabular osteotomy) tend to be young with relatively few comorbidities. For this reason, the operation is usually very well tolerated, and patients return to function soon after the procedure.

8.2 Total hip arthroplasty

According to the American Academy of Orthopaedic Surgeons (AAOS), total hip arthroplasty (THA) is one of the most successful procedures in all of medicine [36]. Over 300,000 THAs are performed yearly in the U.S. Hip osteoarthritis and total hip arthroplasty play a very prominent role in the burden of orthopaedic procedures performed each year worldwide. With the population of the planet ageing at the rate it is, this demand will only increase. Kurtz et al. projected this increased demand in their 2007 paper. It was estimated that by 2030, the demand for primary total hip arthroplasty will rise by 174% to 572,000. Demand for revision THA is expected to double by the year 2026 [37]. These figures confirm that total hip arthroplasty is an essential operation and will only be increasing in the future.

The NICE guidelines published in 2014 suggest appropriate referral requirements for potential hip replacement candidates. Taken directly from the document entitled 'Osteoarthritis: Care and Management', we consider a few recommendations from the section entitled 'Referral for consideration of joint surgery' [38]:

- 1.6.3 Consider referral for joint surgery for people with osteoarthritis who experience joint symptoms (pain, stiffness and reduced function) that have a substantial impact on their quality of life and are refractory to non-surgical treatment. **[2008, amended 2014]**

- 1.6.4 Refer for consideration of joint surgery before there is prolonged and established functional limitation and severe pain. **[2008, amended 2014]**

- 1.6.5 Patient-specific factors (including age, sex, smoking, obesity and comorbidities) should not be barriers to referral for joint surgery. **[2008, amended 2014]**

In 1979, Sir John Charnley, a British Orthopaedic surgeon published his seminal work "Low friction arthroplasty of the hip". In his writings he explained the technique of the total hip arthroplasty. At the time, Charnley was aware of the concepts of friction and how it was important to reduce wear in the implants. He designed a component known as the Charnley stem. This was a monoblock device, meaning it had no modularity or changeable parts. The head size was 22.225 mm in diameter and the bearing surface used for the acetabular replacement was Teflon (polytetrafluoroethylene). Both the femoral and acetabular components were fixed with cement that secured the prostheses in bone. Unfortunately, and understandably with the development of a new technology, there were some issues with the original design of this implant. In the following 40 years, the total hip arthroplasty has evolved significantly in several areas that we will discuss here.

8.2.1 Approach

There are many surgical approaches to hip joint were described. Traditionally, the most common were the anterolateral approach and the posterior approach.

Disadvantages of the anterolateral approach included compromise of the abductor mechanism. Gluteus medius and minimus are traversed in this approach. Although they are repaired afterward, there is often a notable limp or 'Trendelenburg gait' due to abductor weakness. The advantage of this approach is the relative stability it ensures. Historically, the anterolateral approach was associated with a lower risk of dislocation when compared to the posterior approach to the hip. In 1982, the postoperative dislocation rate of the posterior approach was reported as significantly higher when compared to the anterolateral approach. The dislocation rate was reported as 2.3% through the anterolateral approach and 5.8% through the posterior approach [39]. Techniques have advanced since then and the posterior approach has been optimised. Historically, the posterior elements were not always repaired with meticulous technique. In an attempt to reduce the dislocation rate through the posterior approach, posterior soft tissue repair of the capsule and short external rotators has improved the postoperative stability levels to such a degree that surgical approach no longer plays a role in postoperative surgical dislocation rates [40].

8.2.2 Fixation methods

There are two methods of securing the femoral and acetabular components. They may be fixed with cement or with an uncemented technique. Discussion continues regarding the ideal combination of cement and uncemented techniques on both the acetabula side and femoral side of the THA. Options now include fully cemented, fully uncemented, hybrid (cemented stem and uncemented cup) and reverse hybrid (uncemented stem and cemented cup).

Bone cement consists of polymethylmethacrylate. This is a polymer that comes as a liquid (containing the monomer N,N-dimethyltoluidine and hydroquinone) and a powder (consisting of PMMA copolymer, barium dioxide for radio-pacification and benzoyl peroxide for polymerisation initiation). These 2 substances are mixed, and an exothermic chemical reaction ensues. Cement is inserted at around 2–4 minutes and is completely hard at 10–12 minutes. This allows some finesse of the implant position up to a certain point, but beyond that if the final position is suboptimal, all the cement must be removed, which is a significant undertaking in a primary THA.

There are some concerns with the use of cement however. Bone cement implantation syndrome is a characterised by hypotension, hypoxemia, cardiac arrhythmias and cardiac arrest or a combination of any of these [41]. In their study, Ereth et al. assessed this phenomenon prospectively in 35 patients undergoing cemented and uncemented THA with transoesophageal echocardiography and invasive haemodynamic monitoring. Findings confirmed that the use of cement in THA increased the risk of embolisation, reduced cardiac output, increased pulmonary artery pressure and increased pulmonary vascular resistance [41]. This syndrome has also been associated with sudden intraoperative death. The pathology behind this serious complication involves dissemination of bone marrow debris and amorphous cement particles into the circulation which eventually locate in the pulmonary vasculature causing the above described effect [42]. Cemented procedures take a few minutes longer while waiting for the cement to set. Uncemented stems also work on a principle of preserving bone stock whereas cemented stems often remove more cancellous bone stock than their uncemented counter parts. This is important in revision surgery where inadequate bone stock may dictate the usage of a more complex implant and procedure to attain adequate fixation.

Uncemented femoral stems and acetabular components function through a completely different mechanism. By reaming the acetabulum to a certain diameter or broaching the femur to a certain size and then inserting a cup or femoral

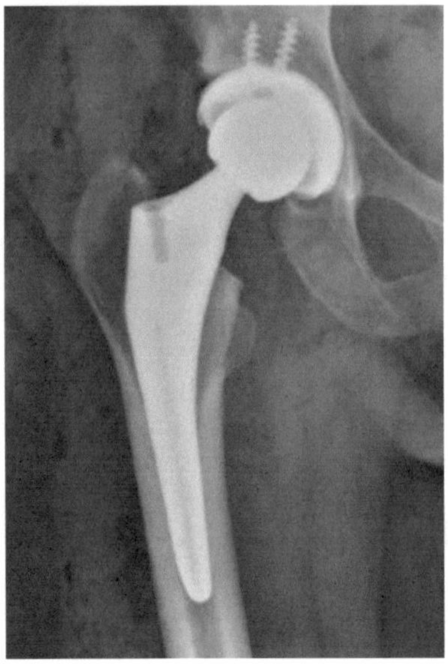

Figure 4.
Uncemented femoral prosthesis.

component that is slightly larger in diameter or size, one can achieve a "press-fit" (**Figure 4**). This provides immediate mechanical stability until biological fixation occurs. Uncemented prosthesis has a porous coating which allows either ingrowth or ongrowth of the native bone. Hydroxyapatite coatings allow growth of bone into metal which provides the fixation in the long term. There is a vogue for using these stems in the younger population as it is necessary to have a reasonable bone stock. There are many reports conferring improved survival of uncemented stems in the younger populations [43]. The risks of bone loss are reportedly higher in the cemented stems and aseptic loosening has also been reported as higher in the cemented stems [44, 45]. There is an increased rate of usage of uncemented stems in modern day practice [46]. Uncemented stems are not without complication however. Many studies have shown that intraoperative periprosthetic fracture rate is higher with the uncemented stem prostheses [34, 47]. Added to this, registry data from around the world has often reported an improved all-cause revision rate in cemented stems over uncemented stems [48, 49]. For this reason, there is no consensus on which stem type is better. The likelihood is that there is a role for both stem types, uncemented in a younger cohort with good bone stock and cemented for a more elderly population with poor bone quality.

8.2.3 Bearing surfaces

The traditional bearing surfaces consisted of a metal femoral head (usually cobalt chrome) and a polyethylene acetabular cup (ultra-high molecular weight polyethylene—UHMWPE). This is a very commonly used combination today. Other surface bearings include ceramic on polyethylene, ceramic on ceramic and metal on metal. Metal on metal bearings have been associated with high failure rates [50]. They have been associated with high levels of adverse reactions to metal debris (ARMD). These local reactions lead to the formation of painful pseudotumours and pain with a difficult revision procedure to correct. High systemic levels of circulating cobalt and chromium may pose a serious health risk to patients. For this reason these implants have fallen out of favour. Ceramic on ceramic bearings have the lowest coefficient of friction and produce the least amount of wear particles which is desirable to reduce the incidence of aseptic loosening. Unfortunately, because these bearings are very rigid, cases of femoral head fracture and squeak have been reported [51].

Ceramic on polyethylene bearings appear to be the most favourable when considering revision rates controlled for bearing surfaces. The New Zealand registry data from 2017 supports this claim also [52]. It is reasonable to conclude that either a ceramic on polyethylene or a metal on polyethylene bearing should be used in modern day total hip arthroplasty. Metal femoral heads are much cheaper than the ceramic options and so arguments for their usage are still valid.

8.3 Revision total hip arthroplasty

The demand for total hip arthroplasty revision will increase significantly in the near future [37]. Large collections of data known as registries now exist and allow analysis on a large scale of the reasons for failure of THA. The National Joint Registry (NJR) is the UK which has the largest collection of THA data in the world every year. According to their 2017 figures, the commonest reasons for revision of 85,199 total hip replacement, in order of decreasing frequency are as follows [53]:

1. Aseptic loosening (41,077)
2. Pain (17,231)
3. Lysis (13.194)
4. Implant wear (11,808)
5. Dislocation/subluxation (11,172)
6. Periprosthetic fracture (8079)
7. Infection (7832)
8. Adverse reaction to metal debris (7095)
9. Malalignment (4448)
10. Implant fracture (2862)
11. Head-socket size mismatch (628)
12. Other (6399)

In order to deal with the above complications, we must improve our technology continually. Developments in the polyethylene have produced new highly-crosslinked polyethylene (XLPE) and vitamin-E treated polyethylene. XLPE has been associated with lower revision rates for aseptic loosening [54]. Vitamin E is an antioxidant which has been shown to reduce wear rates also in the polyethylene [55]. Dislocation rates may be improved through the use of larger femoral heads, restoring length and offset and meticulous surgical repair of the anatomical exposure, regardless of the approach [56]. Periprosthetic fractures are going to rise in the future populations also. General bone health in the elderly population and safe mobilisation will reduce the rates seen. Regarding infection, Parvizi has carried out extensive research in the field. The first definition of prosthetic joint infection (2011) was only described in 2011 [57]. Currently, the 2014 modified accepted definition of PJI is as follows [58]:

A. *There is a sinus tract communicating with the prosthesis, OR*

B. *A phenotypically identical pathogen is isolated by culture from 2 or more separate tissue or fluid samples obtained from the affected prosthetic joint, OR*

C. *When three of the following five criteria exist:*

   i. *Elevated serum erythrocyte sedimentation rate AND serum C-reactive protein concentration*

   ii. *Elevated synovial white blood cell count, OR ++ change on leukocyte esterase test strip*

   iii. *Elevated synovial polymorphonuclear percentage*

   iv. *Positive histological analysis of periprosthetic tissue*

   v. *A single positive culture*

The gold standard treatment for PJI is a 2-stage revision procedure. This involves removal of all infected tissue and insertion of an antibiotic-impregnated spacer (**Figure 5**). This remains in place until the infection has completely cleared. Usually at around 3 months, the second stage procedure is performed. Recurrence rates with this 2-stage approach are much lower when compared with a single stage revision for infection [59]. Clearly, there are many improvements that must be made to reduce the rate of revision THA surgery. This will be an ongoing effort in the future.

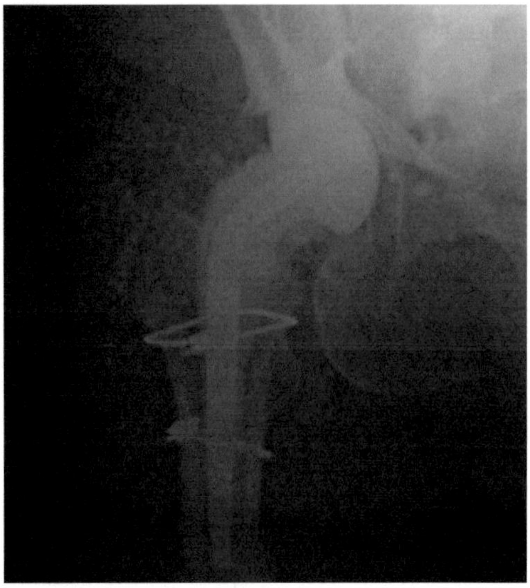

Figure 5.
Antibiotic impregnated spacer with antibiotic beads in the soft tissues.

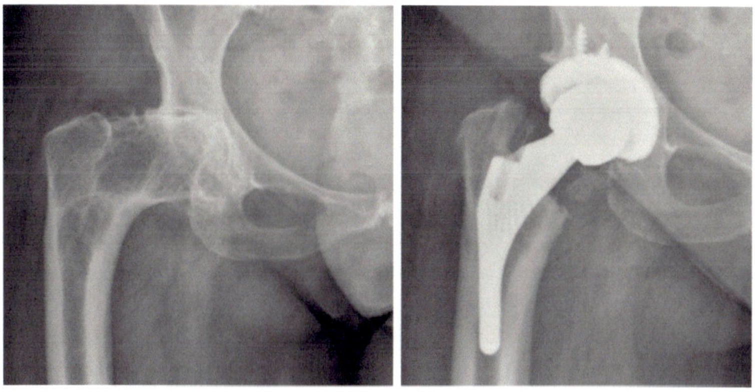

Figure 6.
CAD CAM prosthesis illustrating good fixation in the presence of a highly deformed proximal femur.

8.4 Salvage

Historically, hip arthrodesis and excision hip arthroplasty with complete excision of the femoral head were used to treat end-stage hip osteoarthritis. Hip arthrodesis is rarely indicated anymore due to the success of modern implants. Excision arthroplasty however, does have a role. It may be particularly useful as a salvage procedure in patients with intractable infection. Mobility and pain may be significantly improved through this procedure. Specialised custom-made prostheses which are computer-assisted design and computer assisted manufacture (CAD CAM) have a very niche role in patients with very abnormal hip morphology that cannot be accounted for by standard prostheses (**Figure 6**).

9. Conclusion

Osteoarthritis of the hip is a highly prevalent condition that will be more common in future generations due to the relative increase in the population. As always, history and examination supplemented by good radiographic techniques will guide further management. Total hip arthroplasty is one of the great medical success stories throughout history. There is still room to refine our techniques and this will be the focus of technological advance in the future.

Author details

Gerard A. Sheridan* and James P. Cashman
Cappagh National Orthopaedic Hospital, Dublin, Ireland

*Address all correspondence to: sheridga@tcd.ie

References

[1] Varacallo M, Varacallo M, Johanson NA. Hip, Replacement. Treasure Island (FL): Stat Pearls; 2018

[2] Yu D, Peat G, Bedson J, Jordan KP. Annual consultation incidence of osteoarthritis estimated from population-based health care data in England. Rheumatology (Oxford, England). 2015;**54**(11):2051-2060

[3] Pollard TC, Batra RN, Judge A, Watkins B, McNally EG, Gill HS, et al. Genetic predisposition to the presence and 5-year clinical progression of hip osteoarthritis. Osteoarthritis and Cartilage. 2012;**20**(5):368-375

[4] Miller MD, Thompson. Miller's Review of Orthopaedics. 7th ed. Amsterdam: Elsevier; 2016

[5] Glyn-Jones S, Palmer AJ, Agricola R, Price AJ, Vincent TL, Weinans H, et al. Osteoarthritis. Lancet. 2015;**386**(9991): 376-387

[6] Ramachandran M. Basic Orthopaedic Sciences: The Stanmore Guide. Boca Raton: CRC Press; 2006

[7] Giannoudis PV, Kontakis G, Christoforakis Z, Akula M, Tosounidis T, Koutras C. Management, complications and clinical results of femoral head fractures. Injury. 2009; **40**(12):1245-1251

[8] Magala M, Popelka V, Bozik M, Heger T, Zamborsky V, Simko P. Conservative treatment of acetabular fractures: Epidemiology and medium-term clinical and radiological results. Acta Chirurgiae Orthopaedicae et Traumatologiae Cechoslovaca. 2015; **82**(1):51-60

[9] Galicia K, Thorson C, Banos A, Rondina M, Hopkinson W, Hoppensteadt D, et al. Inflammatory biomarker profiling in Total joint arthroplasty and its relevance to circulating levels of Lubricin, a novel proteoglycan. Clinical and Applied Thrombosis/Hemostasis. 2018;**24**(6): 950-959. DOI: 10.1177/1076029618765090. Epub 2018 Apr 22

[10] Liu J, Khalil RA. Matrix metalloproteinase inhibitors as investigational and therapeutic tools in unrestrained tissue remodeling and pathological disorders. Progress in Molecular Biology and Translational Science. 2017;**148**:355-420

[11] Zhang L, Ma S, Su H, Cheng J. Isoliquiritigenin inhibits IL-1beta-induced production of matrix metalloproteinase in articular chondrocytes. Molecular Therapy—Methods & Clinical Development. 2018; **9**:153-159

[12] Mitchell N, Shepard N. Healing of articular cartilage in intra-articular fractures in rabbits. The Journal of Bone and Joint Surgery American Volume. 1980;**62**(4):628-634

[13] Shapiro F, Koide S, Glimcher MJ. Cell origin and differentiation in the repair of full-thickness defects of articular cartilage. The Journal of Bone and Joint Surgery American Volume. 1993;**75**(4):532-553

[14] Venn M, Maroudas A. Chemical composition and swelling of normal and osteoarthrotic femoral head cartilage. I. Chemical composition. Annals of the Rheumatic Diseases. 1977;**36**(2):121-129

[15] Hilton J. Rest and Pain: A Course of Lectures on the Influence of Mechanical and Physiological Rest in the Treatment of Accidents and Surgical Diseases, and the Diagnostic Value of Pain. London: Bell and Daldy; 1891

[16] Jeanmaire C, Mazieres B, Verrouil E, Bernard L, Guillemin F, Rat AC. Body

composition and clinical symptoms in patients with hip or knee osteoarthritis: Results from the KHOALA cohort. Seminars in Arthritis and Rheumatism. 2018;**47**(6):797-804

[17] Pulos NMM, Courtney PM, Lee GC. Revision THA in obese patients is associated with high re-operation rates at short-term follow-up. The Journal of Arthroplasty. 2014;**29**(9):209-213

[18] Rondon AJ, Tan TL, Schlitt PK, Greenky MR, Phillips JL, Purtill JJ. Total joint arthroplasty in patients with Parkinson's disease: Survivorship, outcomes, and reasons for failure. The Journal of Arthroplasty. 2018;**33**(4): 1028-1032

[19] El Bitar YF, Stone JC, Jackson TJ, Lindner D, Stake CE, Domb BG. Leg-length discrepancy after total hip arthroplasty: Comparison of robot-assisted posterior, fluoroscopy-guided anterior, and conventional posterior approaches. American Journal of Orthopedics (Belle Mead, N.J.). 2015; **44**(6):265-269

[20] Sharma H. FRCS (Tr&Orth) Part II Examination: How to Get Slick in the Clinicals: FRCSOrthExam Education; 2008.

[21] Mao Y, Yu D, Xu C, Liu F, Li H, Zhu Z. The fate of osteophytes in the superolateral region of the acetabulum after total hip arthroplasty. The Journal of Arthroplasty. 2014;**29**(12):2262-2266

[22] Tsurumoto TSK, Okamoto K, Imamura T, Maeda J, Manabe Y, Wakebe T. Periarticular osteophytes as an appendicular joint stress marker (JSM). Analysis in a contemporary Japanese skeletal collection. PLoS One. 2013;**8**(2):e57049

[23] Terjesen T, Gunderson RB. Radiographic evaluation of osteoarthritis of the hip: An inter-observer study of 61 hips treated for late-detected developmental hip dislocation. Acta Orthopaedica. 2012; **83**(2):185-189

[24] Sharma L. Osteoarthritis year in review 2015: Clinical. Osteoarthritis and Cartilage. 2016;**24**(1):36-48

[25] Svege I, Nordsletten L, Fernandes L, Risberg MA. Exercise therapy may postpone total hip replacement surgery in patients with hip osteoarthritis: A long-term follow-up of a randomised trial. Annals of the Rheumatic Diseases. 2015;**74**:164-169

[26] Bennell KL, Egerton T, Martin J, Abbott JH, Metcalf B, McManus F, et al. Effect of physical therapy on pain and function in patients with hip osteoarthritis: A randomized clinical trial. Journal of the American Medical Association. 2014;**311**(19):1987-1997

[27] Organization WH. Cancer pain relief: With a guide to opioid availability. 1986

[28] Strand V, Simon LS, Dougados M, Sands GH, Bhadra P, Breazna A, et al. Treatment of osteoarthritis with continuous versus intermittent celecoxib. The Journal of Rheumatology. 2011;**38**(12):2625-2634

[29] Nakata K, Hanai T, Take Y, Osada T, Tsuchiya T, Shima D, et al. Disease-modifying effects of COX-2 selective inhibitors and non-selective NSAIDs in osteoarthritis: A systematic review. Osteoarthritis and Cartilage. 2018;**26**(10):1263-1273. DOI: 10.1016/j.joca.2018.05.021. Epub 2018 Jun 8

[30] McCabe PS, Maricar N, Parkes MJ, Felson DT, O'Neill TW. The efficacy of intra-articular steroids in hip osteoarthritis: A systematic review. Osteoarthritis and Cartilage. 2016; **24**(9):1509-1517

[31] Chambers AW, Lacy KW, Liow MHL, Manalo JPM, Freiberg AA, Kwon

YM. Multiple hip intra-articular steroid injections increase risk of periprosthetic joint infection compared with single injections. The Journal of Arthroplasty. 2017;**32**(6):1980-1983

[32] Keeney JA, Peelle MW, Jackson J, Rubin D, Maloney WJ, Clohisy JC. Magnetic resonance arthrography versus arthroscopy in the evaluation of articular hip pathology. Clinical Orthopaedics and Related Research. 2004;**429**:163-169

[33] Kemp JL, MacDonald D, Collins NJ, Hatton AL, Crossley KM. Hip arthroscopy in the setting of hip osteoarthritis: Systematic review of outcomes and progression to hip arthroplasty. Clinical Orthopaedics and Related Research. 2015;**473**(3):1055-1073

[34] Aaboud M, Aad G, Abbott B, Abdinov O, Abeloos B, Abidi SH, et al. Search for dark matter produced in association with a Higgs boson decaying to bb[over] using 36 fb^{−1} of pp collisions at sqrt[s]=13 TeV with the ATLAS detector. Physical Review Letters. 2017;**119**(18):181804

[35] Clohisy JC, Beaule PE, O'Malley A, Safran MR, Schoenecker P. AOA symposium. Hip disease in the young adult: Current concepts of etiology and surgical treatment. The Journal of Bone and Joint Surgery American Volume. 2008;**90**(10):2267-2281

[36] Surgeons AAoO. 2015. Available from: https://orthoinfo.aaos.org/en/treatment/total-hip-replacement/

[37] Kurtz S, Ong K, Lau E, Mowat F, Halpern M. Projections of primary and revision hip and knee arthroplasty in the United States from 2005 to 2030. The Journal of Bone and Joint Surgery American Volume. 2007;**89**(4):780-785

[38] nice.org.uk. Osteoarthritis: Care and management clinical guideline [CG177] February 2014

[39] Woo RY, Morrey BF. Dislocations after total hip arthroplasty. The Journal of Bone and Joint Surgery American Volume. 1982;**64**(9):1295-1306

[40] Jameson SS, Baker PN, Mason J, Gregg PJ, Brewster N, Deehan DJ, et al. The design of the acetabular component and size of the femoral head influence the risk of revision following 34 721 single-brand cemented hip replacements: A retrospective cohort study of medium-term data from a National Joint Registry. The Journal of Bone and Joint Surgery British Volume. 2012;**94**(12):1611-1617

[41] Ereth MHWJ, Abel MD, Lennon RL, Lewallen DG, Ilstrup DM, Rehder K. Cemented versus noncemented total hip arthroplasty–embolism, hemodynamics, and intrapulmonary shunting. Mayo Clinic Proceedings. 1992;**67**(11):1066-1074

[42] Razuin R, Effat O, Shahidan MN, Shama DV, Miswan MF. Bone cement implantation syndrome. The Malaysian Journal of Pathology. 2013;**35**(1):87-90

[43] Wechter J, Comfort TK, Tatman P, Mehle S, Gioe TJ. Improved survival of uncemented versus cemented femoral stems in patients aged < 70 years in a community total joint registry. Clinical Orthopaedics and Related Research. 2013;**471**(11):3588-3595

[44] Dan D, Germann D, Burki H, Hausner P, Kappeler U, Meyer RP, et al. Bone loss after total hip arthroplasty. Rheumatology International. 2006;**26**(9):792-798

[45] Eskelinen A, Remes V, Helenius I, Pulkkinen P, Nevalainen J, Paavolainen P. Total hip arthroplasty for primary osteoarthrosis in younger patients in the Finnish arthroplasty register. 4,661 primary replacements followed for 0-22 years. Acta Orthopaedica. 2005;**76**(1):28-41

[46] Lehil MS, Bozic KJ. Trends in total hip arthroplasty implant utilization in the United States. The Journal of Arthroplasty. 2014;**29**(10):1915-1918

[47] Lindberg-Larsen M, Jorgensen CC, Solgaard S, Kjersgaard AG, Kehlet H, Lundbeck Foundation Centre for Fast-Track H, et al. Increased risk of intraoperative and early postoperative periprosthetic femoral fracture with uncemented stems. Acta Orthopaedica. 2017;**88**(4):390-394

[48] Hughes RE, Batra A, Hallstrom BR. Arthroplasty registries around the world: Valuable sources of hip implant revision risk data. Current Reviews in Musculoskeletal Medicine. 2017;**10**(2): 240-252

[49] Hailer NP, Garellick G, Karrholm J. Uncemented and cemented primary total hip arthroplasty in the Swedish hip arthroplasty register. Acta Orthopaedica. 2010;**81**(1):34-41

[50] Maurer-Ertl W, Friesenbichler J, Holzer LA, Leitner L, Ogris K, Maier M, et al. Recall of the ASR XL head and hip resurfacing systems. Orthopedics. 2017; **40**(2):e340-e3e7

[51] Pomeroy E, Rowan F, Masterson E. Atraumatic fracture of a BIOLOX Delta ceramic femoral head articulating with a polyethylene liner: A case report. JBJS Case Connector. 2015;**5**(4):e112

[52] Sharplin PWM, Rothwell A, Frampton C, Hooper G. Which is the best bearing surface for primary total hip replacement? A New Zealand joint registry study. Hip International. 2018; **28**(4):352-362. DOI: 10.5301/hipint.5000585. Epub 2017 Jan 12

[53] Reito A, Lehtovirta L, Lainiala O, Makela K, Eskelinen A. Lack of evidence-the anti-stepwise introduction of metal-on-metal hip replacements. Acta Orthopaedica. 2017; **88**(5):478-483

[54] Callary SA, Solomon LB, Holubowycz OT, Campbell DG, Munn Z, Howie DW. Wear of highly crosslinked polyethylene acetabular components. Acta Orthopaedica. 2015; **86**(2):159-168

[55] van der Veen HC, van den Akker-Scheek I, Bulstra SK, van Raay JJ. Wear, bone density, functional outcome and survival in vitamin E-incorporated polyethylene cups in reversed hybrid total hip arthroplasty: Design of a randomized controlled trial. BMC Musculoskeletal Disorders. 2012;**13**:178

[56] Rowan FE, Benjamin B, Pietrak JR, Haddad FS. Prevention of dislocation after total hip arthroplasty. The Journal of Arthroplasty. 2018;**33**(5):1316-1324. DOI: 10.1016/j.arth.2018.01.047. Epub 2018 Mar 7

[57] Parvizi J, Zmistowski B, Berbari EF, Bauer TW, Springer BD, Della Valle CJ, et al. New definition for periprosthetic joint infection: From the workgroup of the musculoskeletal infection society. Clinical Orthopaedics and Related Research. 2011;**469**(11):2992-2994

[58] Proceedings of the international consensus meeting on periprosthetic joint infection. Foreword. Journal of Orthopaedic Research. 2014;**32** (Supp. 1):S2-S3

[59] Aggarwal VK, Rasouli MR, Parvizi J. Periprosthetic joint infection: Current concept. Indian Journal of Orthopaedics. 2013;**47**(1):10-17

Chapter 3

Contemporary Non-Surgical Considerations in the Management of People with Extra- and Intra-Articular Hip Pathologies

Fiona Dobson, Kim Allison, Laura Diamond and Michelle Hall

Abstract

The hip joint can often be affected by extra- and intra-articular pathologies including gluteal tendinopathy, femoroacetabular impingement syndrome and hip osteoarthritis. Understanding alterations associated with these pathologies will provide greater insight into developing and optimising patient specific treatments. A number of biomechanical and neuromuscular impairment are associated with Femoracetabular impingement (FAI), gluteal tendinopathy (GT) and hip osteoarthritis (OA) conditions including but not limited to muscle weakness, altered postural control, restricted range of motion and altered tendon/joint loading. These alterations can present differently in sub-groups of patients and result directly from the pathological process and/or indirectly from pain and its consequences (e.g. reduced activity). These impairments are often targets for conservative interventions but there is currently little clinical trial evidence to show that treatments can modify these impairments. Clinical trial evidence does, however, support conservative treatment options for each of the pathologies reviewed. Clinical outcome tools used to evaluate the effects of treatment and track change over time are recommended.

Keywords: hip osteoarthritis, femoroacetabular impingement, gluteal tendinopathy, exercise, biomechanics, outcome measurement

1. Introduction

This chapter will present contemporary conservative considerations for the management of extra- and intra-articular hip pathologies including gluteal tendinopathy (GT), femoroacetabular impingement (FAI) syndrome and hip osteoarthritis (OA). The clinical presentation of hip pathology is frequent and can be complex. Over the past decade research has uncovered new insights into biomechanical alterations associations with GT, FAI and hip OA that enables clinicians to better understand the condition and management options. We provide an overview of the most significant discoveries as well as unpack the evidence for effective conservative management. Clinical outcome tools used to evaluate the effectiveness of treatments and track change over time in these hip conditions are reviewed.

IntechOpen

2. Gluteal tendinopathy

Gluteal tendinopathy, also referred to as "greater trochanteric pain syndrome", is a chronic, debilitating musculoskeletal condition affecting the tendinous insertion of the gluteus medius and/or minimus muscles at or above their attachments into the greater trochanter of the femur [1]. The hallmark features of this extra-articular hip condition are pain and tenderness to palpation at or around the region of the greater trochanter [1–3]. Prevalence rates of GT have been reported at 18% of those aged 50–79 years presenting to general practitioners [3]. Individuals with GT are most frequently over the age of 40 years [4] and typically experience pain during walking, stair climbing and/or lying on the affected side [1–3].

2.1 Biomechanical considerations in gluteal tendinopathy

2.1.1 Important anatomical and biomechanical considerations

The trochanteric bursae were previously considered the primary structure implicated in greater trochanteric pain [5]. However, new evidence from magnetic resonance imaging (MRI) [6, 7], ultrasound [8, 9] and surgical case series' [7, 10] has led to a contemporary understanding of the pathological mechanisms of the gluteal tendons underpinning greater trochanter pain. This progressive understanding of tendon involvement has necessitated important advances regarding biomechanical considerations associated with GT.

The gluteal tendons are vulnerable to anatomical compression against the (i) underlying greater trochanter, as they wrap over the borders of its bony facets into their respective insertions [11], and (ii) from the overlying iliotibial band (ITB), particularly as the hip moves into adduction. With increasing adduction of the femur relative to the pelvis, the insertion of the gluteus minimus and medius muscles on the greater trochanter are moved away from their respective origins on the ilium, placing longitudinal tensile and transverse tensile strain through the tendon fibres passing over the greater trochanter. In addition, the ITB exerts progressively higher compressive forces at the greater trochanter as the hip moves into hip adduction (4 N at 0°, increased by nine-fold to 36 N at 10° and 106 N at 40°) [12], which has direct consequences for gluteal tendon loading. Excessive tensile and compressive loads are accepted to be detrimental for tendon health and particularly relevant for the development and perpetuation of tendinopathy [13]. Thus, dynamic control of hip adduction is pertinent in the assessment and management of GT [14].

2.1.2 Hip abductor muscle weakness and clinical relevance to loading biomechanics

Like other tendinopathies, muscle weakness is a feature of GT [15]. Strength deficiencies of 32% of the hip abductor muscles on the symptomatic hip and 23% on the asymptomatic hip have been identified in individuals with clinically and MRI diagnosed GT compared to age- and sex-comparable controls [15]. The primary functional role of the hip abductor muscles is to maintain alignment of the pelvis in the frontal plane during gait, to eccentrically control the provocative position of hip adduction [16]. The relationship between hip adduction angle and hip abductor tendon loading in GT highlights the importance of abductor muscle strength for adequate eccentric control of hip adduction in this patient group [16]. Clinicians often evaluate hip abductor function by visually evaluating a patient's ability to maintain and control position of the pelvis in single leg stance (SLS) [17]. Further, SLS kinematics are considered relevant for control of single leg loading during gait.

Data from three-dimensional motion capture analysis identified that individuals with GT exhibit greater lateral pelvic shift and hip adduction in preparation for SLS, and more hip adduction and less contralateral pelvic elevation during SLS in the frontal plane when compared to age and sex matched controls [18] (**Figure 1**). Though these findings may be, in part, explained by hip abductor muscle weakness [18], they also provide important insight into why single leg stance is provocative for many individuals with GT. Specifically, the increased potential tensile and compressive load through the gluteal tendons as the muscles work to control the position of the pelvis on the femur, is a likely relevant mechanism for tendon overload and pain.

2.1.3 Gait biomechanics

To date, only one study has evaluated *walking* kinematics and kinetics in individuals with GT compared to healthy controls. In contrast to pain-free controls, individuals with GT exhibit a significantly greater external hip adduction moment during the stance phase of walking [19] and during *stair climbing* [20]. These observations are thought to have distinct clinical relevance, given the external hip adduction moment represents an internal hip abductor moment contributed to by active and passive tension in the primary hip abductor muscles (i.e. the gluteus minimus and medius) [21]. Of importance to clinicians who use visual observation as part of their assessment in GT, contralateral pelvic drop is associated with a greater magnitude of the external hip adduction moment [19]. While data has shown that individuals with GT exhibit greater contralateral pelvic drop during late stance compared to controls, with implications for hip adduction angles and tendon loading, this between-group difference during walking was small on average (1.4 degrees), with questionable clinical relevance [19]. This small mean difference may be explained by variation in walking strategies utilised by participants in the GT group. A secondary analysis identified distinct subgroups in those with GT [19]. This novel and clinically relevant observation highlights that people with GT can compensate for hip abductor weakness in different ways, which coincide with compensations reported in individuals with intra-articular hip pain [22] and

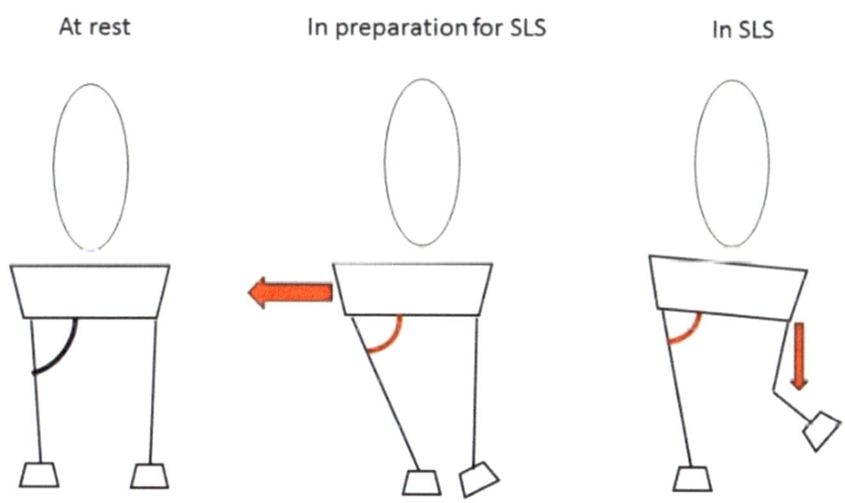

Figure 1.
In preparation for single leg stance (SLS) individuals with gluteal tendinopathy exhibit greater lateral pelvic shift over the stance limb (and subsequently greater hip adduction angle) and maintain a position of single leg stance with greater contralateral pelvic drop (and subsequently hip adduction angle).

with extra-articular hip pathology, such as GT [19]. Specifically, two subgroups were identified in those with GT: (1) individuals demonstrating an uncompensated Trendelenburg (contralateral pelvic drop and associated contralateral trunk lean where no compensation is made for hip abductor weakness and the position of the pelvis cannot be maintained in the frontal plane); and (2) individuals demonstrating a compensated Trendelenburg (ipsilateral trunk lean in an attempt to bring the centre of mass closer to the base of support, resulting in reduced hip abductor muscle requirements and maintenance of the position of the pelvis in the frontal plane) (**Figure 2**).

2.2 Non-surgical management for gluteal tendinopathy

Evidence for the management of gluteal tendinopathy is continuing to emerge. Historically, as a result of limited understanding of the pathology and associated impairments in GT, treatment had been simplistic, targeting symptoms or the presumed pathological involvement of the trochanteric bursae. More recently, drawing from contemporary evidence in other tendinopathies and an understanding of tendon structure and function, exercise interventions for GT have been refined and are beginning to be tested in randomised controlled trials with promising results. The most recent systematic review at the time of print concluded that poor quality and insufficient data prevented any conclusions to be drawn regarding optimal treatment for greater trochanteric pain syndrome including GT [23]. Studies in this review and others describe interventions of surgical tendon repair, ITB release and bursectomy, corticosteroid injection, home exercise, shock wave therapy and dry needling [23]. Issues arise when interpreting the collective results of these studies with respect to GT, as the samples are diverse with respect to co-morbidities (e.g. hip OA, lumbar pathology), symptom duration, and most importantly, clinical and

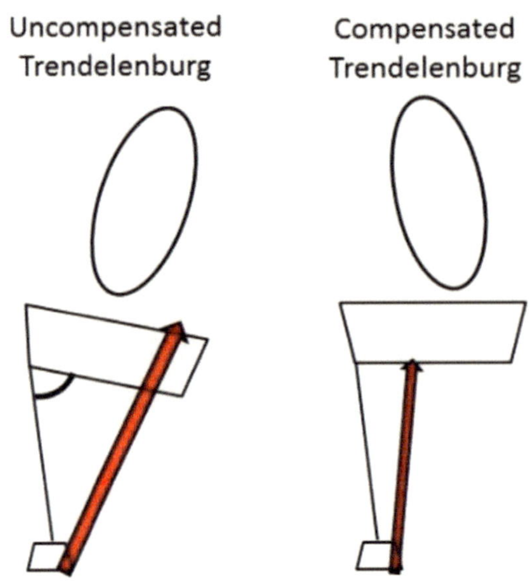

Figure 2.
Subgroups have been identified in individuals with gluteal tendinopathy during walking [19]. Some individuals walk with an uncompensated Trendelenburg (contralateral pelvic drop and trunk lean, increasing the centre of mass from the hip joint centre and subsequently influencing the magnitude of the external adduction moment), while some adopt a compensated Trendelenburg (ipsilateral trunk lean, bringing the centre of mass closer to the hip joint centre, a strategy to reduce the magnitude of the external hip adduction moment and requirement for the hip abductor muscles, maintaining alignment of the pelvis in the frontal plane).

imaging diagnosis specific to GT. Further, very few interventions have been evaluated in randomised controlled trials.

The strong focus on corticosteroid injection in GT arises from the original theory that trochanteric pain was due to an inflammatory process within the trochanteric bursae. However, the effectiveness and safety of the use of corticosteroid injection in tendinopathy is debatable. Evidence from a high quality systematic review pooling 41 studies evaluating the effect of corticosteroid injection on upper limb, patella and Achilles tendinopathies suggests that while cortisone improves symptoms in the short term, there are no long term effects at 13–26 weeks or ≥ 52 weeks [24]. While these findings cannot be directly inferred to GT, a similar attenuation effect of symptom relief in response to corticosteroid injection has been demonstrated in three clinical trials in greater trochanteric pain syndrome [25–27], questioning the efficacy of corticosteroid use in GT.

Given that tendon is a metabolically active tissue that maintains its integrity in response to tensile loading, exercise and load modification appear to be important aspects of effective treatment in management of tendinopathy [28]. In order to modify tendon load in the lower limb, addressing lower limb biomechanics and neuromuscular control is considered an effective clinical strategy [14]. Specific to GT, modifying compressive load at the greater trochanter is thought to be particularly relevant [5, 27]. *Load modification* can be achieved my reducing time spent in sustained positions of hip adduction where the gluteal tendons are vulnerable to compressive loading against the greater trochanter below and iliotibial band above (e.g. sitting cross legged, standing 'hanging on one hip', sleeping on the affected side or the unaffected side with the affected limb crossing into hip adduction) or dynamic adduction during gait [14]. The latter is thought to be best achieved by including (1) *functional weight bearing hip abductor muscle exercises* (e.g. bridging, squat, side-stepping) *focusing on pelvic alignment control* in the frontal and transverse planes double to single leg loading and by focusing on (2) *hip abductor strengthening exercises* to address muscle weakness and increase loading capacity of the gluteal tendons [15] (e.g. side-stepping with band, reformer based sliders). A fundamental principle in tendinopathy management which must be applied in this exercise prescription context is that of *progressive graduated overload* to enable tendon remodelling and adaptation [14]. It is essential that exercise difficulty is gradually increased as tolerated to ensure optimal muscle activation to enable gains in muscle strength and function without significant aggravation of pain. Finally specific to the context of GT, (3) *motor control of the entire hip abductor muscle mechanism* thought to be important to reduce overactivity of tensor fascia lata (and subsequent ITB tension) relative to the deeper segments of the gluteus minimus and medius muscles [29] to facilitate gluteal tendon tensile loading and avoid compressive loads, known to be detrimental to tendon health. Patient tactile feedback over the tensor fascia lata and gluteal muscles is thought to be a useful clinical strategy to address this goal [14].

A recent clinical trial demonstrated that a progressive exercise program incorporating functional training, targeted strengthening and dynamic motor control of the pelvis, delivered with patient education over 8-weeks under supervision of a physiotherapist, was superior to a wait-and-see approach or corticosteroid injection [27]. These results are promising and contribute to the body of evidence for treatment of GT. Importantly, they also add to the contemporary conversation that emphasises the need for patient education in management. As outlined, it is evident that hip abductor muscle strength, biomechanical and neuromuscular patterns be considered in the assessment and management of GT. However, data from individuals with GT highlights that the kinematic presentation of GT is heterogeneous [19, 20]. Thus a 'one size fits all' approach to assessment and management is unlikely to be effective. Clinicians should evaluate patients who present with GT with respect to specific biomechanical and neuromuscular impairments, and tailor treatment and load modification based on the principles of tendinopathy treatment.

3. Femoroacetabular impingement syndrome

FAI syndrome is a motion related condition of the hip joint and is associated with hip pain and impaired function in younger active adults [30]. FAI is characterised by abnormally shaped hip bones (i.e. head of femur and/or acetabulum), which can lead to mechanical impingement during movement [30]. Repetitive mechanical impingement is thought to lead to chondral stresses that cause irreversible structural pathology [31]. FAI syndrome is considered a principal determinant of future development of hip osteoarthritis [32].

3.1 Biomechanical considerations in femoroacetabular impingement syndrome

3.1.1 Hip joint biomechanics

Evidence for altered hip joint biomechanics during movement in individuals with FAI syndrome is mounting [33]. Gait has been well studied in this population. Findings from systematic reviews [31, 33] and empirical studies provide moderate evidence for less sagittal plane hip range of motion (ROM) [34], primarily driven by a lower peak hip extension angle [35], during gait in individuals with FAI syndrome compared to healthy controls. Lower peak hip internal rotation angle [35, 36] and lower peak hip external rotation joint torque [35] have also be reported during stance in FAI syndrome compared to healthy controls. However, the biomechanical adaptations exhibited by individuals with FAI syndrome during gait are generally small on average, and consequently of uncertain clinical significance.

Hip joint biomechanics during squatting [37–39] in FAI syndrome also differs only subtly from individuals without pain or FAI morphology. Though some studies report that individuals with FAI syndrome are unable to squat as deep as controls [37, 39], hip flexion range is not significantly reduced during task completion [37–39]. Individuals with FAI syndrome place the hip in a more adducted position during squatting [38] and step ascent [40], which may be secondary to hip abductor muscle weakness commonly reported in FAI syndrome cohorts [41]. Biomechanical comparisons during these more demanding tasks targeting positions of impingement (i.e. squatting and step ascent) have extended knowledge regarding altered hip joint biomechanics in individuals with FAI syndrome. Nevertheless, the implications of these alterations, including any relationship with pain and/or function and/or joint structure remain unclear.

3.1.2 Biomechanics of adjacent segments

Individual variation in movement strategy and interaction between adjacent body segments (i.e. pelvis, trunk) may account for the small between-group differences observed in hip joint biomechanics when comparing individuals with FAI syndrome to healthy controls. Failure to consider such factors may explain the modest effects of conservative treatment [42] and the unrestored hip function observed post-operatively [36]. Reduced sagittal plane pelvis range of motion has been identified during squatting in FAI syndrome compared to healthy controls

[39], and has been proposed as a risk factor for symptom presentation [43]. Greater anterior pelvic tilt has also been reported in FAI syndrome during squatting [37] and step descent [44] compared to healthy controls. This biomechanical alteration may be counterproductive for pathology since an increase in anterior pelvic position will promote hip flexion and thus impingement.

Few studies have considered pelvic and trunk control in the frontal plane despite the implications for hip joint loading [45]. Control of frontal plane pelvic alignment during single leg support is necessary to prevent movement into impingement. Pain and/or hip abductor muscle weakness, both features of FAI syndrome, could hinder control of the pelvis in the frontal plane. On the other hand, altered frontal plane control of the trunk may moderate provocative hip joint contact forces (i.e. reduced demand on hip abductor muscles), and has been observed in cohorts with hip osteoarthritis [22, 46]. Recent findings from a step ascent task corroborate that control of adjacent segments may play an important role in symptom management in FAI syndrome [40]. When individuals with FAI syndrome were sub-grouped based on trunk and pelvis dominant strategies, those who exhibited lateral trunk lean and maintained neutral pelvis alignment reported no pain and prevented the hip from moving towards an impinging position. It is reasonable to suggest that this strategy may alleviate load on the abnormal hip joint structures. In direct contrast to this, 86% of participants who exhibited poor pelvis control, inherently moving the hip into an impinging position, reported moderate levels of pain [40]. Control of—and interaction between—adjacent body segments may play an important role in symptomatic and structural preservation or deterioration in FAI syndrome. Further, altered hip joint function remains unresolved post-operatively [36], suggesting that a hip-only treatment focus may be misguided. Functional biomechanics is modifiable, and could be changed by conservative interventions and rehabilitation programs [47].

3.1.3 Patient subgrouping

FAI syndrome is a complex condition [48] with no common pathological pathway [30]. Patient presentation is heterogeneous, which may explain the modest treatment effects [42]. Different biomechanical strategies are used by separate subgroups of participants to perform a task [38, 49], albeit some more advantageous than others for symptoms and function. As with established hip OA [50], no conservative treatment is likely to be effective for all individuals with FAI syndrome. Maximum efficacy will only be attained with interventions catered to the individual. More research must be done to improve understanding of the patient-specific biomechanical alterations associated with FAI syndrome in order to better manage the disease and its consequences.

3.1.4 Implications for joint structure

Biomechanical alterations in individuals with FAI syndrome are subtle but may relate to enhanced protection for the hip, albeit with possible long-term consequences. It comes as no surprise that individuals with FAI syndrome exhibit less prominent biomechanical alterations than individuals with structural damage and hip OA [51]. Individuals with FAI syndrome have less severe morphological deformities and accordingly, exhibit more subtle biomechanical modifications. The absence of longitudinal studies means that it is not known whether these small biomechanical alterations are precursors to the larger deviations observed in those with established hip OA.

3.2 Non-surgical management for femoroacetabular impingement syndrome

Arthroscopic hip surgery is the most common treatment for FAI syndrome [52]. Despite a dramatic upsurge in the number of surgeries performed over the past decade [52], surgical intervention for FAI syndrome does not completely restore hip joint function to that of healthy controls [36] or uniformly improve pain [53], despite correction of the hip's bony abnormalities. This may be because surgery corrects the local mechanical issue (i.e. correction of the bony abnormalities until impingement free motion is obtained), but without resolution of the altered movement strategies adopted pre-operatively.

Findings from the only large randomised controlled trial comparing hip arthroscopy and best conservative care for the treatment of FAI syndrome support the short-term efficacy of arthroscopic hip surgery [54]. However, patients in both groups reported significant improvements in hip-related quality of life at 12-months, and the costs associated with surgery were higher than with conservative care [54]. Non-surgical treatments for FAI syndrome, such as exercise, activity adaptation and education, are globally recommended [48], and attractive given the relatively low harmful risks and associated costs. Identification of non-surgical interventions to reduce the burden of hip OA in its early stages, including FAI syndrome, is an important public health priority [55]. At present, conservative treatment effects for FAI syndrome are also modest [42, 56], likely due, in part, to a lack of understanding regarding the underlying mechanisms associated with clinical and structural decline.

3.2.1 Conservative care

Theoretically, an adequately designed, evidence-based, appropriately administered conservative management program may have the potential to alleviate symptoms, and in turn prevent disease progression, thus postponing or negating the need for surgery [56]. Current clinical practice entails combinations of physiotherapist-led rehabilitation, education, and activity modification for the management of FAI syndrome [48, 56]. There is little evidence from randomised control trials to guide conservative care for FAI syndrome, which means that conservative treatments are largely based on clinical theory and/or extrapolation of evidence from other clinical conditions.

Potential targets for conservative treatment include the abnormal movement patterns and hip muscle weakness seen in patients with FAI syndrome [31]. Gait assessment alone is unlikely to provide clear information to guide treatment of FAI syndrome. However, the biomechanical alterations at the hip joint and adjacent segments apparent during more demanding tasks (e.g. squatting, step ascent and descent) may be relevant in the clinical management of this patient population. Altered movement patterns in the form of altered hip joint biomechanics have been identified during tasks with similar demands in these patients post-operatively [36]. Pre-operative treatments addressing these biomechanical abnormalities may also have scope to improve surgical outcomes.

Retraining of deep hip muscle function (e.g. quadratus femoris, obturator internus) is a common objective of non-operative management [57] and post-operative rehabilitation [58] for FAI syndrome. Conservative care commonly targets deep hip external rotator muscle strengthening and neuromuscular retraining with the aim of improving dynamic hip joint stability [57]. Although experimental evidence suggests that activation of these deep muscles may contribute to dynamic stability in a healthy hip [59], it is less clear if adaptations in neuromuscular control are associated with FAI syndrome. Cross-sectional data acquired during gait provide preliminary evidence of the extent and nature of FAI-related changes to deep hip muscle activation [49]. However, an improved understanding of deep hip muscle function during more demanding, provocative tasks is needed to provide a comprehensive recommendation for retraining.

Hip strength assessment may be important in the clinical management of FAI syndrome. Evaluation of agonist/antagonist and/or between-limb strength ratios could be particularly beneficial clinically, as body size normalisation and control normative data for individual movement directions are not required. Reduced abduction strength in FAI patients [41] may have important implications as the abductor muscles control the position of the pelvis relative to the femur [60]. This is critical to prevent movement (i.e. contralateral pelvic drop) into a position that impinges the hip joint during single leg weight bearing tasks, such as those commonly required in sport where FAI syndrome has been identified (e.g. soccer, dancing, football) [61]. Treatment programs targeting the primary abductor muscles may improve pelvic-femoral stability during single leg task performance in individuals with FAI syndrome, though any implications of such treatments for symptoms and joint structure are not yet clear.

3.2.2 Optimising treatment

Clinical interventions to restore normal musculoskeletal function around the hip joint may be beneficial, but future research is needed to determine whether these features can and should be changed, and whether this improves outcomes. Cam impingement has been proposed as a modifiable risk factor for hip OA [32]. Optimising treatments relies on the identification of novel treatment targets to slow femoral lesion progression and prolong the development of structural damage and early hip OA.

A critical step in the clinical management of individuals with FAI syndrome is to identify which biomechanical and neuromuscular features are: (i) positive and should be encouraged; (ii) negative and should be discouraged; and (iii) potentially positive prior to surgery to compensate for the abnormal morphology but should be a target for treatment following surgery to prevent further impairments. It would be precipitous to categorise these features without the support of longitudinal data. Nevertheless, it is abundantly clear that the widespread implications for FAI-related clinical practice depend on the appropriate classification of any modifiable targets for treatment.

The evaluation of conservative management programs, that include a range of techniques to modify joint motion/loading/function such as joint mobilisation techniques, hip bracing, and targeted exercise programs (including range of motion, strengthening, and/or neuromuscular retraining) are required on a range of outcomes in FAI syndrome (including any modifiable risk factors). Though the evidence underpinning these treatments is still in its infancy, the development of conservative treatments, including post-operative rehabilitation strategies and pre-operative training programs that aim to improve surgical outcomes, is a critical component as we move towards improving treatment outcomes.

4. Hip osteoarthritis

Hip OA is a major public health problem and affects one in four adults over their lifetime [62]. The condition substantially impairs quality of life and causes pain and physical dysfunction. Around the world, hip replacement surgery for hip OA is on the rise, and the burden of OA on society and health care cost will continue to rise due to the ageing population and escalation in obesity rates [63]. Therefore, treatments that reduce symptoms and delay the need for joint replacement are critical.

4.1 Biomechanical considerations in hip osteoarthritis

Kinematic and kinetic alterations are reported in people with hip OA compared to healthy controls. There is marked interest in hip joint loading as a culprit for disease progression, arguably due to the evidence in knee OA. Higher knee joint loading has been implicated in structural joint degeneration in middle-aged people at risk of early knee OA [64] and in individuals with established with knee OA [65]. However, few longitudinal studies have evaluated the association between hip joint biomechanics during gait and alterations in hip joint structure [66, 67]. A 12-month longitudinal study of women concluded that higher cumulative hip joint loading assessed as the number of steps per day, in the frontal plane, was associated with joint space narrowing at the hip joint [67]. However, there is insufficient evidence regarding which direction of loading magnitude change is detrimental for joint health (i.e. under- or over-loading). Recent investigations have highlighted the effect of sex, stage of disease and symptom severity on measures of joint loading, as well as the intricate relationships between these measures and hip joint load. Similar to other hip pathologies, hip OA is a heterogeneous disease, and exploration of patient and disease characteristics are needed to better understand moderators of *hip joint load*, a potential disease modifier. For the clinician, 'joint loading' is not examinable or visible in the clinical setting. However, the trunk and pelvis, together are major contributors to the centre of mass, the position of which (relative to the hip joint centre) influences hip joint loading. Thus, visual examination of trunk and pelvic kinematics during functional tasks is an important part of assessment.

4.1.1 Sex and joint loading

Measures of frontal plane loading appear to be dependent on sex. For example, in disease-free individuals the external hip adduction moment is typically greater in females as compared to males [68]. Between-sex differences in anatomy may explain these differences, at least in part. Females typically have a wider pelvis than males [69], which inherently increases the lateral distance of the centre of mass from the hip joint centre, and thus increases the hip adduction moment. However, any underlying anatomical differences appear secondary to disease stage when explaining difference in frontal plane moments. A series of cross-sectional studies indicate that between-sex differences in frontal plane loading are apparent in those with unilateral mild-to-moderate hip OA [70], while measures of hip joint loading are not different between men and women with end-stage hip OA [68]. The indirect effect of sex on hip joint loading earlier in the disease process was also detected in meta-regression analysis of a systematic review. Studies with a greater proportion of men demonstrated a greater average standardised mean difference for reduced frontal plane loading between people with hip OA compared to controls [71]. Given that loading may be relevant for disease progression, it may be clinically pertinent to consider sex-specific interventions for hip OA.

4.1.2 Stage of disease and joint loading

Measures of hip joint loading are also dependent on disease severity. A recent systematic review and meta-analysis of 13 studies suggests that people with hip OA appear to underload compared to controls [72]. Moreover, the sub-group analysis indicates that people awaiting total hip replacement (i.e. greater disease severity) underload the hip joint compared to controls; whereas people with less severe disease have comparable measures of joint loading in the sagittal and frontal plane [73]. These observations are consistent with empirical investigations determining the influence of disease severity on measures of hip joint loading [71]. Understanding the effect of joint loading on joint structure and symptoms is imperative to guide conservative hip OA management.

4.1.3 Relevance of pain and symptoms

Slow walking speed is a risk factor for mortality [74] and chronic functional limitation in older adults [75]. A systematic review of 17 studies estimated that people with hip OA have a self-selected walking speed of 0.95 m/s, a markedly 26% slower than controls [76]. In light of critical walking speed estimates of 1.0 m/s [72], the observation that people with hip OA walk slower than critical walking speed estimates is alarming. Slower walking speed can be attributable to symptoms and a reduction in stride length in people with hip OA [76]. However, a recent cross-sectional study [73] investigating people with moderate radiographic hip OA with and without symptoms found that irrespective of symptoms, people with radiographic hip OA walk slower than disease-free individuals. These data question symptoms as a cause for reduced walking speed and instead, appear to reflect a longer-term adaptation hip joint degeneration. In addition to being an important marker of function [74, 75], walking speed also influences measures of hip joint loading. Investigators grapple with understanding whether alteration in measures of joint loading are predominately reflections of alterations in walking speed [77]. It appears that in addition to slower walking speed, neuromuscular adaptations are likely to underpin the reduction in hip joint loading in individuals with hip OA.

Evidence regarding pain during walking and how it influences movement strategies is emerging in OA literature [78]. In hip OA, the overall evidence supports the contention that people with hip OA, particularly at end-stage of the disease, underload during walking compared to controls [79]. The premise being that symptoms potentially cause people to walk slower. However, recent cross-sectional findings refute this logic [72], highlighting the complexities between symptoms and joint loading. In a study of people with unilateral mild-to-moderate radiographic hip OA, those who reported moderate pain during walking had higher frontal plane joint loading compared to people who reported less pain during walking [72]. These data suggest that people with mild or no pain during walking modified their gait biomechanics to exert lower frontal hip joint loading. Evidently, the relationship between symptoms and joint loading is intricate.

4.2 Conservative management for hip osteoarthritis

"*What can I do myself to decrease OA symptoms and prevent the OA from getting worse?*" These were prioritised as the most important questions by patients and health professionals in relation to hip and knee OA [80]. Treatments to reduce hip OA symptoms and delay the need for joint replacement are critical. Joint replacement is costly and is only reserved for end-stage disease when non-surgical treatments are no longer effective. Current clinical guidelines [55, 81, 82], including the recent update by the Royal Australian College of General Practitioners [83], emphasise that a healthy lifestyle consisting of regular exercise and weight management are the core management strategies for hip OA. Interestingly, there are no clinical trials for weight management in people with hip OA [83], and consequently the subsequent overview explores evidence for exercise in these individuals.

Exercise is advised for all people with hip OA irrespective of age, disease severity, symptoms and co-morbidities [81]. A recent meta-analyses in people with hip OA identified 12 RCTs and showed small-to-modest beneficial effects of exercise on pain (standardised mean difference [SMD] −0.28, 95% CI: −0.45 to −0.10) and physical function (−0.34 SMD, 95% CI: −0.50 to −0.18) compared to no exercise [84]. Notably, two trials including 154 people scheduled for total hip replacement [85, 86], had large improvements in pain (−0.63 SMD, 95% CI: −0.95 to −0.30) and physical function (−0.71 SMD, 95% CI: −1.04 to −0.39) following 8–10 weeks of exercise. In addition to beneficial effects on symptoms, exercise can potentially delay total hip replacement. A long-term follow-up of a clinical trial found that exercise combined with patient education can potentially reduce the need for total hip replacement by 44% in people with hip OA [87].

Evidence strongly supports the use of exercise as treatment for hip OA symptoms and can potentially prevent disease progression. In line with high quality evidence and clinical guidelines, physiotherapists in the UK [88] and Australia [89] typically recommend exercise in the management of hip OA. However, knowledge on the specifics of exercise prescription is a recognised barrier to exercise uptake [90]. Reintahl [91] eloquently likens exercise prescription to drug prescription. For example, the physician determines the type of medication, the amount or intensity, the frequency of intake and the duration of use. Exercise prescription typically follows the frequency, intensity, type, time, volume and progression (FITT-VP) principles [92], but evidence on best exercise prescription is lacking for treatment of hip OA symptoms. Below, we provide an update on the current evidence for dosage and type of exercise.

4.2.1 Exercise dosage

Meta-analyses from trials with high compliance to the American College of Sports Medicine (ACSM) exercise guidelines with respect to dosage was −0.42 SMD (95% CI: −0.58 to −0.26) for pain, and studies with uncertain compliance to ACSM dosage was −0.05 SMD (95% CI, −0.35 to −0.25) for pain. Improvement in physical function of −0.41 SMD (95% CI −0.58, −0.24) was comparable to pain in trials with high compliance to the ACSM dosage guidelines while effect from trials with uncertain compliance was −0.23 SMD (95% CI, −0.52, 0.06) [84]. These data support the prescription of exercise in accordance with ACSM guidelines, particularly in relation to pain. A Cochrane review revealed that patients with OA are confused about their cause of pain, and they do not know what they should and should not do, and as a consequence, they avoid activity for fear of causing harm [93]. Collectively, health professionals can use existing evidence to reassure patients about the value of exercise to safely manage symptoms.

4.2.2 Exercise type

All clinical trials to date include lower-limb strengthening [85, 86, 94–103], which is unsurprising given that hip and knee muscle weakness is widely established in people with hip OA [104]. However, only a few clinical trials in people with hip OA include aerobic exercise [96, 101, 103]. People with hip OA often present with co-morbidities, such as poor cardiovascular fitness and low psychological wellbeing, and these are associated with greater hip OA symptom severity [105, 106]. Aerobic exercise and muscle strengthening exercise address different impairments associated with hip OA symptoms and the adaptations people experience are distinctly different for each exercise type. Aerobic exercise may enhance the effects of strengthening exercise on hip OA symptoms by targeting

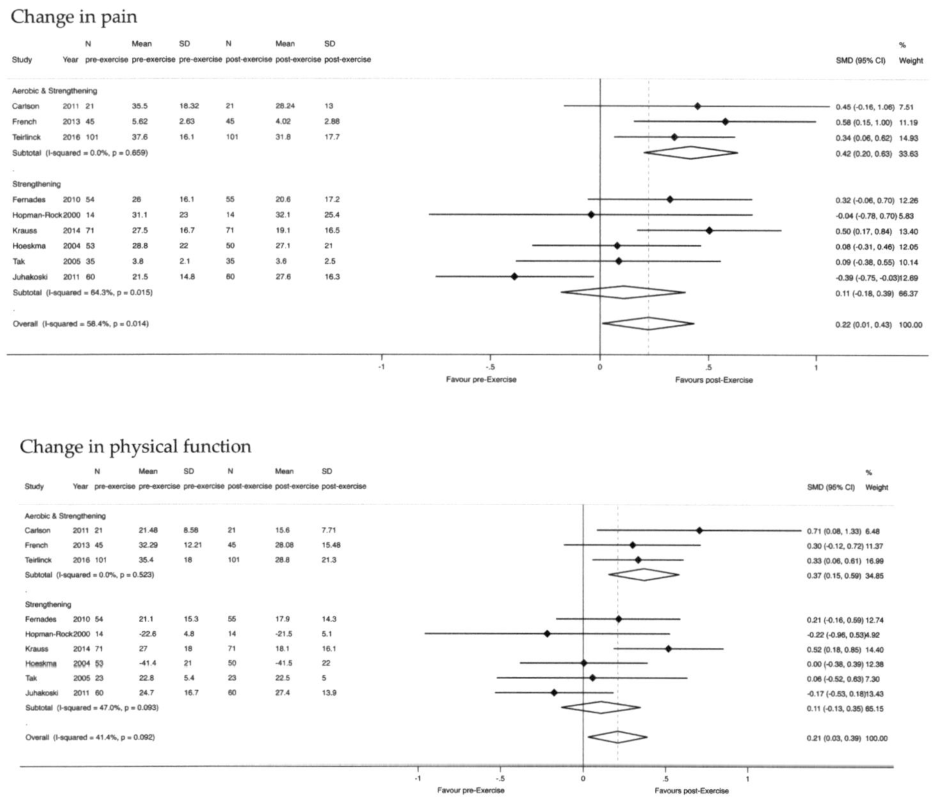

Figure 3.
Change in pain (top plot) and physical function (bottom plot) in people with mild to moderate hip osteoarthritis after a combination of aerobic and strengthening exercise or strengthening exercise alone.

cardiovascular fitness and psychological well-being [107]. In our own analysis, pain and physical function scores before and after exercise interventions in people with mild-to-moderate hip OA were sourced through publications and direct author contact. Changes in pain and physical function in studies that used a combination of aerobic and strengthening exercise are compared to those studies that used strengthening exercise only (**Figure 3**). This preliminary comparison provides support that greater effects on hip OA-related pain and physical dysfunction occur when a combination of aerobic and strengthening exercise is prescribed rather than strengthening exercise alone (**Figure 3**). Despite the clear rationale to support the premise that a combination of aerobic and muscle strengthening exercise could be more beneficial for hip OA symptoms then either exercise on its own, no clinical trials have directly tested this hypothesis.

5. Outcome measures

Measuring patient specific outcomes following an intervention or over a course of care is important for clinical research and best evidence-based practice. Outcomes that are most meaningful from the patient's perspective, such as those that measure symptoms of pain and physical function during activities of daily living, are imperative [108, 109]. Other outcomes of impairments, such as strength, flexibility, range of motion are also important for clinicians and researchers to assess and monitor, but are more often used for clinical differential diagnosis or prognosis and are usually secondary outcome measures to pain and physical function [109–111].

Measurement of pain and physical function are complex and cover multiple dimensions. For example, pain can be measured in multiple contexts including intensity, duration, type and location. Physical functioning can not only be measured in many contexts but it also crosses multiple domains. According to the International Classification of Functioning, Disability and Health (ICF), physical function spans *body functions and structure, activity* and *participation* domains [112].

Many outcome tools for pain and physical function have been described for hip conditions and a selection of tools with the best level of measurement evidence is recommended [109]. Ideally, measure outcomes should be suitably valid, reliable and responsive to change. Known values of the minimum important difference (MID) are important for interpreting meaningful change and are useful to help set individual targets and goals with patients [113].

Patient outcomes can be measured using patient-reported outcome measures (PROMs) and performance-based tests measured by the clinician/researcher. Pain is usually measured with PROMs, such as pain scales and questionnaires, however physical functioning can be measured with both PROMs and performance-based tests. Performance-based tests reflect what patients can do rather than what they think they can do, which is usually captured with PROMs. When assessing physical function, it is recommended that both PROMs and performance-based tests are used as they can encapsulate different information as they test different constructs of function [114].

Patient outcomes can be measured using individual-specific, condition-specific and/or generic outcome tools. There are several condition-generic, individual-specific PROMs that are useful in assessing and monitoring symptoms and function in people with a variety of hip conditions.

5.1 Condition-generic, individual-specific patient-reported outcome measures

The 11-point Numerical Pain Rating Scale (NPRS) can be used to track pain symptoms and can be customised to individual dimensions of pain. For example, average, current or greatest pain in the previous 24-hours or week can be measured ranging from 0 (no pain) to 10 (worst possible pain). Similarly, pain during an activity such as walking can be measured ranging from 0 (no pain on walking) to 10 (severe pain on walking). The MID for the NPRS (scale 0–10) in musculoskeletal conditions ranges from 1.5 points (small change) to 3.5 points (large change) [115] and in hip OA is defined as a change in pain during walking of 1.8 points [116].

The Patient-reported functional scale (PRFS) [117] assesses current level of difficulty associated with 3–5 activities that the individual identifies as being important, each measured on an 11-point scale, where 0 is unable to perform the activity and 10 is able to perform the activity as normal. The MID for the PSFS ranges from 1.3 points (small change) to 2.7 points (large change [115].

Patient-perceived change following an intervention over time can be measured on a Global Rating of Change (GROC) scale, customised to the outcome to be measured, and used by the patient to rate their perceived overall change as worse, no change or better. If worse, the patient is asked to indicate how much worse, from very much worse to slightly worse. If better, then they are asked how much better, from slightly better to very much better. An example is the 11-point GROC [118] with a change scale ranging from −5 to +5. The GROC scale can be very useful to set individual levels of acceptable change over a stated time frame and to set individual treatment goals [119].

There are also several condition-generic PROMs useful for assessing quality of life in a variety of hip conditions. These include the Medical Outcome Study 36 questions short form (SF-36) [120], the EuroQol (EQ-5D) [121] and the Assessment of quality of life (AQOL) [122]. Patient-specific quality of life questionnaires have also been developed for hip OA such as the Osteoarthritis Knee and Hip Quality of Life questionnaire (OAKHQOL) [123].

5.2 Condition-specific outcomes

The following sections will outline condition-specific PROMs and performance-based tests used to measure pain and physical function in the hip conditions outlined previously in this chapter. Outcomes are selected based on available clinical practice guideline recommendations, measurement property evidence and reported use within clinical trials. A summary of the outcomes presented across the three hip conditions including the outcome domains, scoring method, and where known, MID values are provided in **Table 1**.

5.2.1 Gluteal tendinopathy

A number of valid and reliable measures used in recent clinical trials to measure change in pain and function in patients following corticosteroid injections and exercise [129] and recommended in a systematic review [130] are promising suitable outcomes for people with gluteal tendinopathies. These include the Victorian Institute of Sport Assessment-Gluteal tendon (VISA-G) questionnaire [131] that evaluates the severity of disability using 8 items about current pain and function. Regarding performance-based tests, the single-leg stance test with light fingertip support is useful to assess provocation of pain during a 30-second period. A report of pain over the greater trochanteric region indicates a positive test. This test has excellent sensitivity (100%) and specificity (97.3%), making it an ideal screening out test when pain is negative [2]. Additionally, the pain-free time and the time the patient can maintain a level pelvis in single-leg stance can also be recorded to measure change over time. Other performance-based tests include the single leg squat test where the ability to single leg squat as far as possible 5 times with the non-support leg out front and arms folded across the chest is rated on 5 criteria as good, fair or poor [132] and the star-excursion balance test that evaluates the ability to stand on one leg and reach the other leg into eight directions as far as possible [133].

5.2.2 Femoroacetabular impingement

A number of specifically designed, reliable and well-validated PROMs are recommended for measuring outcomes in people with FAI by an international, multidisciplinary consensus statement endorsed by 25 clinical societies worldwide [48]. The International Hip Outcome Tool (iHOT-33) is a patient-derived questionnaire designed to measure hip-related quality of life in young adults with non-arthritic hip pain over four domains: symptoms and functional limitations; sports and recreational physical activities; job related concerns; and social, emotional and lifestyle concerns [124]. The hip and groin outcome score (HAGOS) was developed for physically active young to middle-aged adults [134] and contains 37 questions, covering six domains of pain; symptoms; physical function in daily living, sport and recreation; participation in physical function, sports and recreation, and hip and/or groin related QOL. The hip outcome score (HOS) [126] was developed to assess treatment outcomes of hip arthroscopy in young to middle-aged individuals and contains 28 questions, covering activities of daily living, and sport.

	Condition	Outcome	Items	Scoring	MID
Patient-reported outcomes					
Numeric Pain Rating Scale (NPRS)	All	Pain	1	0–10 scale Higher scores indicate worst pain	1.5–3.5 points in musculoskeletal conditions [115]; 1.8 points for hip OA [116]
Patient-Specific Functional Scale (PSFS)	All	Physical function	3–5	0–10 scale Higher scores indicate higher function	1.3–2.7 points in musculoskeletal conditions [115]
Global Rating of Change (GROC) Scale	All	Change in condition	1	Variable scales e.g. −5 to +5, higher scores indicate improvement	Individualised e.g. moderately better/ somewhat worse
Victorian Institute of Sport Assessment-Gluteal tendon (VISA-G)	GT	Pain, physical function	8	0–100 mm VAS Higher scores indicate less pain and higher function	
International Hip Outcome Tool (iHOT-33)	FAI	Pain, physical function, quality of life	33	0–100 mm VAS, where 100 indicates better quality of life score	Between 6 mm [124] and 10 mm [125] in young adults after hip arthroscopy
Hip and Groin Outcome Score (HAGOS)	FAI	Pain, physical function, quality of life	37	0–100 mm VAS where 100 indicates no problems	Less than 10 mm (10%) on each subscale in young adults after hip arthroscopy [125]
Hip Outcome Score (HOS)	FAI	Physical function	28	0–100 mm VAS Higher scores on each subscale indicates higher levels of physical function	5-9 mm for ADL subscale; 6 mm for sports subscale in young adults after arthroscopic surgery [125, 126]
Western Ontario and McMaster Universities Osteoarthritis Index (WOMAC)	Hip OA	Pain, stiffness, physical function	32	0–4 point scale Higher scores on each of subscale indicate greater disability.	6/68 points on the physical function subscale in people with hip OA [127]
Hip disability and Osteoarthritis Outcome Score (HOOS)	Hip OA	Pain, physical function, quality of life	40	0–4 point scale where 0 indicates extreme symptoms and 4 indicates no symptoms	

	Condition	Outcome	Items	Scoring	MID
Performance-based tests					
30-sec single leg stance	GT	Pain, physical function	1	Pain free; hold pelvis level up to 30 s	
Single leg squat test	GT	Physical function	1	Rated as good, fair, poor	
Star-excursion balance test	GT	Physical function, balance	1	Distance reached in centimetres normalised to leg length with larger distances indicating greater balance and higher physical function	
Stair Climb test	All	Physical function	1	Faster time in seconds indicates higher level of physical function	
30-sec chair stand test	Hip OA	Physical function	1	Great number of repetitions indicates higher level of physical function	2–3 repetitions in people with hip OA [128]
40-m fast paced walk test	Hip OA	Physical function	1	Faster time in seconds or greater speed in metres/second indicates higher level of physical function	0.2–0.3 m/s in people with hip OA [128]
Timed Up and Go test	Hip OA		1	Faster time in seconds indicates higher level of physical function	0.8–1.4 s in people with hip OA [128]
6-minute walk test	Hip OA	Physical function, aerobic capacity	1	Greater distance covered in metres indicates higher level of physical function and aerobic capacity	

ADL, activities of daily living; FAI, femoroacetabular impingement; MID, minimum important difference; OA, osteoarthritis; VAS, visual analogue scale.

Table 1.
Patient-reported outcome measures and performance-based tests for hip conditions.

A clear recommendation of which performance-based tests should be used for this condition is yet to be made, however tests that are reliable and best discriminate between individuals with FAI and those without have been described [135]. This includes the 5-times sit-to-stand test where the time taken to transition from sitting to standing from a standard chair five times is recorded in seconds; and the stair ascend test where the time taken to ascend a flight of stairs as quickly as possible without using a handrail is recorded in seconds.

5.2.3 Hip osteoarthritis

Numerous clinical practice guidelines, for example [83, 108, 111], and recommendations, for example [110, 136, 137] informed from high level measurement property evidence and expert consensus strongly recommend a number of condition-specific PROMs. The Western Ontario and McMaster Universities Osteoarthritis (WOMAC) Index [138] measures pain, stiffness and physical function The Hip disability and Osteoarthritis Outcome Score (HOOS) [139] consists of five subscales; pain, other symptoms, function in daily living, function in sport and recreation, and hip related quality of life. This scale incorporates items from the WOMAC scale so can also be extracted from this questionnaire.

The Osteoarthritis Research Society International (OARSI) recommend performance-based measures of physical function representing typical activities relevant to individuals diagnosed with hip or knee OA [136, 137]. Comprehensive descriptions, including set up, equipment, preparation (environment, participant, and tester), procedures, verbal instructions and scoring are available on the OARSI website: http://oarsi.org/research/physical-performance-measures along with videos of each recommended test. The full set includes five tests and the first three were recommended as the minimum core set: (i) *30 s chair stand test* where the number of full stands a person can perform in a 30 s period is recorded in seconds; (ii) *40 m fast-paced walk test* where the time taken to walk 4 × 10 m as quickly but as safely as possible is recorded in seconds which can be converted to speed recorded in metres per second; (iii) *stair climb test* where the time taken to ascend and descend a flight of stairs (with optional use of handrail) is recorded in seconds; (iv) *timed up and go* where the time taken to stand up from a standard chair with arm-rests, walk at regular pace to a line 3 m away, turn around and return to the seated position is recorded in seconds; and (v) *six-minute walk test* where the maximum possible distance walked in 6 min is recorded in metres covered.

6. Conclusion

Evidence supports exercise as a promising solution to the most important questions asked by patients with extra- and intra-articular hip pathologies and health professionals. Exercise can reduce hip symptoms and potentially prevent disease progression. Stakeholders, including but not limited to, health care professionals, research communities, consumer organisations, and local and national policy makers must make a deliberate effort to translate the positive message of exercise as a treatment for hip conditions. Research is ongoing to further empower patients and clinicians with evidence around best-prescription for exercise.

Author details

Fiona Dobson[1*], Kim Allison[1], Laura Diamond[2] and Michelle Hall[1]

1 Department of Physiotherapy, Centre for Health, Exercise and Sports Medicine, University of Melbourne, Carlton, Australia

2 School of Allied Health Sciences, Griffith University, Gold Coast, Australia

*Address all correspondence to: fdobson@unimelb.edu.au

References

[1] Fearon AM, Scarvell JM, Neeman T, et al. Greater trochanteric pain syndrome: Defining the clinical syndrome. British Journal of Sports Medicine. 2013;**47**(10):649-653

[2] Lequesne M, Mathieu P, Vuillemin-Bodaghi V, et al. Gluteal tendinopathy in refractory greater trochanter pain syndrome: Diagnostic value of two clinical tests. Arthritis and Rheumatism. 2008;**59**(2):241-246

[3] Segal NA, Felson DT, Torner JC, et al. Greater trochanteric pain syndrome: Epidemiology and associated factors. Archives of Physical Medicine & Rehabilitation. 2007;**88**(8):988-992

[4] Glyn-Jones S, Palmer A, Price A, et al. Osteoarthritis. The Lancet. 2015;**386**(9991):376-387

[5] Grimaldi A, Mellor R, Hodges PW, et al. Gluteal tendinopathy: A review of mechanisms. Assessment and Management. Sports Medicine. 2015;**48**(8):1107-1119

[6] Woodley S, Nicholson H, Livingstone V, et al. Lateral hip pain: Findings from magnetic resonance imaging and clinical examination. Journal of Orthopaedic & Sports Physical Therapy. 2008;**38**(6):313-328

[7] Lequesne M, Djian P, Vuillemin V, et al. Prospective study of refractory greater trochanter pain syndrome. MRI findings of gluteal tendon tears seen at surgery. Clinical and MRI results of tendon repair. Joint, Bone, Spine. 2008;**75**(4):458-464

[8] Long SS, Surrey DE, Nazarian LN. Sonography of greater trochanteric pain syndrome and the rarity of primary bursitis. American Journal of Roentgenology. 2013;**201**(5):1083-1086

[9] Fearon AM, Scarvell JM, Cook JL, et al. Does ultrasound correlate with surgical or histologic findings in greater trochanteric pain syndrome? A pilot study. Clinical Orthopaedics and Related Research. 2010;**468**(7):1838-1844

[10] Domb BG, Carreira DS. Endoscopic repair of full-thickness gluteus medius tears. Arthroscopy Techniques. 2013;**2**(2):e77-e81

[11] Cook JL, Purdam C. Is compressive load a factor in the development of tendinopathy? British Journal of Sports Medicine. 2011;**46**(3):163-168

[12] Birnbaum K, Siebert CH, Pandorf T, et al. Anatomical and biomechanical investigations of the iliotibial tract. Surgical and Radiologic Anatomy: SRA. 2004;**26**(6):433-446

[13] Cook J, Rio E, Purdam C, et al. Revisiting the continuum model of tendon pathology: What is its merit in clinical practice and research? British Journal of Sports Medicine. 2016;**50**(19):1187-1191

[14] Grimaldi A, Fearon AM. Gluteal tendinopathy: Integrating pathomechanics and clinical features in its management. Journal of Orthopaedic & Sports Physical Therapy. 2015;**45**(11):910-922

[15] Allison K, Vicenzino B, Wrigley TV, et al. Hip abductor muscle weakness in individuals with gluteal tendinopathy. Medicine and Science in Sports and Exercise. 2016;**48**(3):346-352

[16] Al-Hayani A. The functional anatomy of hip abductors. Folia Morphologica. 2009;**68**(2):98-103

[17] Grimaldi A. Assessing lateral stability of the hip and pelvis. Manual Therapy. 2011;**16**(1):26-32

[18] Allison K, Bennell KL, Grimaldi A, et al. Single leg stance control in individuals with symptomatic gluteal tendinopathy. Gait & Posture. 2016;**49**:108-113

[19] Allison K, Wrigley TV, Vicenzino B, et al. Kinematics and kinetics during walking in individuals with gluteal tendinopathy. Clinical Biomechanics. 2016;**32**:56-63

[20] Allison K, Vicenzino B, Bennell KL, et al. Kinematics and kinetics during stair ascent in individuals with gluteal tendinopathy. Clinical Biomechanics. 2016;**40**:37-44

[21] Yoon YS, Mansour JM. The passive elastic moment at the hip. Journal of Biomechanics. 1982;**15**(12):905-910

[22] Thurston A. Spinal and pelvic kinematics in osteoarthrosis of the hip joint. Spine. 1985;**10**(5):467-471

[23] Del Buono A, Papalia R, Khanduja V, et al. Management of the greater trochanteric pain syndrome: A systematic review. British Medical Bulletin. 2012;**102**:115-131

[24] Coombes BK, Bisset L, Vicenzino B. Efficacy and safety of corticosteroid injections and other injections for management of tendinopathy: A systematic review of randomised controlled trials. Lancet (London, England). 2010;**376**(9754):1751-1767

[25] Denman M. Corticosteroid injections improved short-term, but not long-term, recovery and pain in the greater trochanteric pain syndrome. Annals of Internal Medicine. 2011;**155**(8)JC4

[26] Rompe JD, Segal NA, Cacchio A, et al. Home training, local corticosteroid injection, or radial shock wave therapy for greater trochanter pain syndrome. American Journal of Sports Medicine. 2009;**37**(10):1981-1990

[27] Mellor R, Bennell K, Grimaldi A, et al. Education plus exercise versus corticosteroid injection use versus a wait and see approach on global outcome and pain from gluteal tendinopathy: Prospective, single blinded, randomised clinical trial. BMJ. 2018;**361**:k1162

[28] Larsson MH, Käll I, Nilsson-Helander K. Treatment of patellar tendinopathy—A systematic review of randomized controlled trials. Knee Surgery, Sports Traumatology, Arthroscopy. 2012;**20**(8):1632-1646

[29] Allison K, Salomoni SE, Bennell KL, et al. Hip abductor muscle activity during walking in individuals with gluteal tendinopathy. Scandinavian Journal of Medicine & Science in Sports. 2018;**28**(2):686-695

[30] Ganz R, Parvizi J, Beck M, et al. Femoroacetabular impingement: A cause for osteoarthritis of the hip. Clinical Orthopaedics and Related Research. 2003;**417**:112-120

[31] Diamond LE, Dobson FL, Bennell KL, et al. Physical impairments and activity limitations in people with femoroacetabular impingement: A systematic review. British Journal of Sports Medicine. 2015;**49**(4):230-242

[32] Agricola R, Heijboer MP, Bierma-Zeinstra SM, et al. Cam impingement causes osteoarthritis of the hip: A nationwide prospective cohort study (CHECK). Annals of the Rheumatic Diseases. 2013;**72**(6):918-923

[33] King MG, Lawrenson PR, Semciw AI, et al. Lower limb biomechanics in femoroacetabular impingement syndrome: A systematic review and meta-analysis. British Journal of Sports Medicine. 2018;**52**(9):566-580

[34] Diamond LE, Wrigley TV, Bennell KL, et al. Hip joint biomechanics during gait in people with and without symptomatic femoroacetabular

impingement. Gait & Posture. 2016;**43**:198-203

[35] Hunt MA, Guenther JR, Gilbart MK. Kinematic and kinetic differences during walking in patients with and without symptomatic femoroacetabular impingement. Clinical Biomechanics (Bristol, Avon). 2013;**28**(5):519-523

[36] Rylander J, Shu B, Favre J, et al. Functional testing provides unique insights into the pathomechanics of femoroacetabular impingement and an objective basis for evaluating treatment outcome. Journal of Orthopaedic Research: Official Publication of the Orthopaedic Research Society. 2013;**31**(9):1461-1468

[37] Bagwell JJ, Snibbe J, Gerhardt M, et al. Hip kinematics and kinetics in persons with and without cam femoroacetabular impingement during a deep squat task. Clinical Biomechanics. 2016;**31**:87-92

[38] Diamond LE, Bennell KL, Wrigley TV, et al. Squatting biomechanics in individuals with symptomatic femoroacetabular impingement. Medicine and Science in Sports and Exercise. 2017;**49**(8):1520-1529

[39] Lamontagne M, Kennedy MJ, Beaule PE. The effect of cam FAI on hip and pelvic motion during maximum squat. Clinical Orthopaedics and Related Research. 2009;**467**(3):645-650

[40] Diamond LE, Bennell KL, Wrigley TV, et al. Trunk, pelvis and hip biomechanics in individuals with femoroacetabular impingement syndrome: Strategies for step ascent. Gait & Posture. 2018;**61**:176-182

[41] Diamond LE, Wrigley TV, Hinman RS, et al. Isometric and isokinetic hip strength and agonist/antagonist ratios in symptomatic femoroacetabular impingement. Journal of Science and Medicine in Sport. 2016;**19**(9):696-701

[42] Reiman MP, Thorborg K. Femoroacetabular impingement surgery: Are we moving too fast and too far beyond the evidence? British Journal of Sports Medicine. 2015;**49**(12):782-784

[43] Ng KC, Lamontagne M, Adamczyk AP, et al. Patient-specific anatomical and functional parameters provide new insights into the pathomechanism of cam FAI. Clinical Orthopaedics and Related Research. 2015;**473**(4):1289-1296

[44] Lewis CL, Loverro KL, Khuu A. Kinematic differences during single-leg step-down between individuals with femoroacetabular impingement syndrome and individuals without hip pain. The Journal of Orthopaedic and Sports Physical Therapy. 2018;**48**(4):270-279

[45] Bergmann G, Deuretzbacher G, Heller M, et al. Hip contact forces and gait patterns from routine activities. Journal of Biomechanics. 2001;**34**(7):859-871

[46] Meyer CAG, Corten K, Fieuws S, et al. Evaluation of stair motion contributes to new insights into hip osteoarthritis-related motion pathomechanics. Journal of Orthopaedic Research. 2015;**34**(2):187-196

[47] Kemp J. Hip-related pain. In: Brukner P, Khan KM, editors. Clinical Sports Medicine. Sydney: McGraw-Hill; 2012. pp. 510-544

[48] Griffin DR, Dickenson EJ, O'Donnell J, et al. The Warwick agreement on femoroacetabular impingement syndrome (FAI syndrome): An international consensus statement. British Journal of Sports Medicine. 2016;**50**(19):1169-1176

[49] Diamond LE, Van den Hoorn W, Bennell KL, et al. Coordination of deep hip muscle activity is altered

in symptomatic femoroacetabular impingement. Journal of Orthopaedic Research. 2017;**35**(7):1494-1504

[50] Driban JB, Sitler MR, Barbe MF, et al. Is osteoarthritis a heterogeneous disease that can be stratified into subsets? Clinical Rheumatology. 2010;**29**(2):123-131

[51] Kumar D, Wyatt C, Chiba K, et al. Anatomic correlates of reduced hip extension during walking in individuals with mild-moderate radiographic hip osteoarthritis. Journal of Orthopaedic Research: Official Publication of the Orthopaedic Research Society. 2015;**33**(4):527-534

[52] Bozic KJ, Chan V, Valone FH 3rd, et al. Trends in hip arthroscopy utilization in the United States. The Journal of Arthroplasty. 2013;**28** (8 Suppl):140-143

[53] Clohisy JC, St John LC, Schutz AL. Surgical treatment of femoroacetabular impingement: A systematic review of the literature. Clinical Orthopaedics and Related Research. 2010;**468**(2):555-564

[54] Griffin DR, Dickenson EJ, Wall PDH, et al. Hip arthroscopy versus best conservative care for the treatment of femoroacetabular impingement syndrome (UK FASHIoN): A multicentre randomised controlled trial. Lancet (London, England). 2018;**391**(10136):2225-2235

[55] Zhang W, Nuki G, Moskowitz RW, et al. OARSI recommendations for the management of hip and knee osteoarthritis: Part III: Changes in evidence following systematic cumulative update of research published through January 2009. Osteoarthritis and Cartilage. 2010;**18**(4):476-499

[56] Wall PD, Fernandez M, Griffin D, et al. Nonoperative treatment for femoroacetabular impingement: A systematic review of the literature. PM & R: The Journal of Injury, Function, and Rehabilitation. 2013;**5**(5):418-426

[57] Kemp JL, Moore K, Fransen M, et al. A phase II trial for the efficacy of physiotherapy intervention for early-onset hip osteoarthritis: Study protocol for a randomised controlled trial. Trials. 2015;**16**:26

[58] Bennell KL, O'Donnell JM, Takla A, et al. Efficacy of a physiotherapy rehabilitation program for individuals undergoing arthroscopic management of femoroacetabular impingement—The FAIR trial: A randomised controlled trial protocol. BMC Musculoskeletal Disorders. 2014;**15**:58

[59] Hodges PW, McLean L, Hodder J. Insight into the function of the obturator internus muscle in humans: Observations with development and validation of an electromyography recording technique. Journal of Electromyography and Kinesiology: Official Journal of the International Society of Electrophysiological Kinesiology. 2014;**24**(4):489-496

[60] Gottschalk F, Kourosh S, Leveau B. The functional anatomy of tensor fasciae latae and gluteus medius and minimus. Journal of Anatomy. 1989;**166**:179-189

[61] Philippon M, Schenker M, Briggs K, et al. Femoroacetabular impingement in 45 professional athletes: Associated pathologies and return to sport following arthroscopic decompression. Knee Surgery, Sports Traumatology, Arthroscopy. 2007;**15**(7):908-914

[62] Murphy LB, Helmick CG, Schwartz TA, et al. One in four people may develop symptomatic hip osteoarthritis in his or her lifetime. Osteoarthritis and Cartilage. 2010;**18**(11):1372-1379

[63] GBD 2016 DALYs and HALE Collaborators. Global, regional, and national disability-adjusted life-years (DALYs) for 333 diseases and injuries and healthy life expectancy (HALE) for 195 countries and territories, 1990-2016: A systematic analysis for the Global Burden of Disease Study 2016. Lancet (London, England). 2017;**390**(10100):1260-1344

[64] Hall M, Wrigley TV, Metcalf BR, et al. Do moments and strength predict cartilage changes after partial meniscectomy? Medicine and Science in Sports and Exercise. 2015;**47**(8):1549-1556

[65] Bennell KL, Bowles KA, Wang Y, et al. Higher dynamic medial knee load predicts greater cartilage loss over 12 months in medial knee osteoarthritis. Annals of the Rheumatic Diseases. 2011;**70**(10):1770-1774

[66] Kumar D, Wyatt C, Lee S, et al. Sagittal plane walking patterns are related to MRI changes over 18-months in people with and without mild-moderate hip osteoarthritis. Journal of Orthopaedic Research: Official Publication of the Orthopaedic Research Society. 2018;**36**(5):1472-1477

[67] Tateuchi H, Koyama Y, Akiyama H, et al. Daily cumulative hip moment is associated with radiographic progression of secondary hip osteoarthritis. Osteoarthritis and Cartilage. 2017;**25**(8):1291-1298

[68] Foucher KC. Sex-specific hip osteoarthritis-associated gait abnormalities: Alterations in dynamic hip abductor function differ in men and women. Clinical Biomechanics (Bristol, Avon). 2017;**48**:24-29

[69] Wang SC, Brede C, Lange, Poster CS, Lange AW, Kohoyda-Inglis C, et al. Gender differences in hip anatomy: Possible implications for injury tolerance in frontal collisions. Annual Proceedings. Association for the Advancement of Automotive Medicine. 2004;**48**:287-301

[70] Allison K, Hall M, Wrigley TV, et al. Sex-specific walking kinematics and kinetics in individuals with unilateral, symptomatic hip osteoarthritis: A cross sectional study. Gait & Posture. 2018;**65**:234-239

[71] Foucher KC. In: Aaron R, editor. Gait Pathomechanics in Hip Disease. Cham: Springer; 2015

[72] Hall M, Allison K, Wrigley TV, et al. Frontal plane hip joint loading according to pain severity in people with hip osteoarthritis. Journal of Orthopaedic Research: Official Publication of the Orthopaedic Research Society. 2018;**36**(6):1637-1644

[73] Hall MCS, Shakoor N, Leurgans SE, Foucher KC. Hip joint loading according to symptoms in people with mild radiographic osteoarthritis. Under revision

[74] Studenski S, Perera S, Patel K, et al. Gait speed and survival in older adults. Journal of the American Medical Association. 2011;**305**(1):50-58

[75] Cesari M, Kritchevsky SB, Penninx BW, et al. Prognostic value of usual gait speed in well-functioning older people—Results from the Health, Aging and Body Composition Study. Journal of the American Geriatrics Society. 2005;**53**(10):1675-1680

[76] Constantinou M, Barrett R, Brown M, et al. Spatial-temporal gait characteristics in individuals with hip osteoarthritis: A systematic literature review and meta-analysis. The Journal of Orthopaedic and Sports Physical Therapy. 2014;**44**(4):291-2B7

[77] Astephen Wilson JL. Challenges in dealing with walking speed in knee osteoarthritis gait analyses. Clinical Biomechanics (Bristol, Avon). 2012;**27**(3):210-212

[78] Boyer KA. Biomechanical response to osteoarthritis pain treatment may impair long-term efficacy. Exercise and Sport Sciences Reviews. 2018;**46**(2):121-128

[79] Diamond LE, Allison K, Dobson F, et al. Hip joint moments during walking in people with hip osteoarthritis: A systematic review and meta-analysis. Osteoarthritis Cartilage. 2018;**26**(11):1415-1424

[80] Claassen A, Kremers-van de K, van den Hoogen FHJ, et al. The most important frequently asked questions of patients with hip or knee osteoarthritis: A best-worst scaling exercise. Arthritis Care & Research (Hoboken). 2018; Jul 28. DOI: 10.1002/acr.23719. [Epub ahead of print]

[81] Fernandes L, Hagen KB, Bijlsma JW, et al. EULAR recommendations for the non-pharmacological core management of hip and knee osteoarthritis. Annals of the Rheumatic Diseases. 2013;**72**(7):1125-1135

[82] National Clinical Guideline Centre. Osteoarthritis. Care and Management in Adults. National Institiute for Health and Care in Excellence [Internet]. 2014

[83] Royal Australian College of General Practitioners. Royal Australian College of General Practitioners. 2nd ed. 2018. Available from: https://www.racgp.org.au/your-practice/guidelines/musculoskeletal/hipandkneeosteoarthritis/

[84] Moseng T, Dagfinrud H, Smedslund G, et al. The importance of dose in land-based supervised exercise for people with hip osteoarthritis. A systematic review and meta-analysis. Osteoarthritis and Cartilage. 2017;**25**(10):1563-1576

[85] Hermann A, Holsgaard-Larsen A, Zerahn B, et al. Preoperative progressive explosive-type resistance training is feasible and effective in patients with hip osteoarthritis scheduled for total hip arthroplasty—A randomized controlled trial. Osteoarthritis and Cartilage. 2016;**24**(1):91-98

[86] Villadsen A, Overgaard S, Holsgaard-Larsen A, et al. Immediate efficacy of neuromuscular exercise in patients with severe osteoarthritis of the hip or knee: A secondary analysis from a randomized controlled trial. The Journal of Rheumatology. 2014;**41**(7):1385-1394

[87] Svege I, Nordsletten L, Fernandes L, et al. Exercise therapy may postpone total hip replacement surgery in patients with hip osteoarthritis: A long-term follow-up of a randomised trial. Annals of the Rheumatic Diseases. 2015;**74**(1):164-169

[88] Holden MA, Bennell KL, Whittle R, et al. How do physical therapists in the United Kingdom manage patients with hip osteoarthritis? Results of a cross-sectional survey. Physical Therapy. 2018;**98**(6):461-470

[89] Cowan SM, Blackburn MS, McMahon K, et al. Current Australian physiotherapy management of hip osteoarthritis. Physiotherapy. 2010;**96**(4):289-295

[90] Dobson F, Bennell KL, French SD, et al. Barriers and facilitators to exercise participation in people with hip and/or knee osteoarthritis: Synthesis of the literature using behavior change theory. American Journal of Physical Medicine & Rehabilitation. 2016;**95**(5):372-389

[91] Reinthal A. Getting the dosage right in balance exercise prescription: The intensity problem. Journal of Novel Physiotherapies. 2017;7:e147

[92] American College of Sports Medicine ACSM's Health-Related Physical Fitness Assessment Manual.

lippincott Williams & Wilkins Philadelphia, USA; 2013

[93] Hurley M, Dickson K, Hallett R, et al. Exercise interventions and patient beliefs for people with hip, knee or hip and knee osteoarthritis: A mixed methods review. The Cochrane Database of Systematic Reviews. 2018;**4**:Cd010842

[94] Abbott JH, Robertson MC, Chapple C, et al. Manual therapy, exercise therapy, or both, in addition to usual care, for osteoarthritis of the hip or knee: A randomized controlled trial. 1: Clinical effectiveness. Osteoarthritis and Cartilage. 2013;**21**(4):525-534

[95] Fernandes L, Storheim K, Sandvik L, et al. Efficacy of patient education and supervised exercise vs patient education alone in patients with hip osteoarthritis: A single blind randomized clinical trial. Osteoarthritis and Cartilage. 2010;**18**(10):1237-1243

[96] French HP, Cusack T, Brennan A, et al. Exercise and manual physiotherapy arthritis research trial (EMPART) for osteoarthritis of the hip: A multicenter randomized controlled trial. Archives of Physical Medicine and Rehabilitation. 2013;**94**(2):302-314

[97] Hoeksma HL, Dekker J, Ronday HK, et al. Comparison of manual therapy and exercise therapy in osteoarthritis of the hip: A randomized clinical trial. Arthritis and Rheumatism. 2004;**51**(5):722-729

[98] Hopman-Rock M, Westhoff MH. The effects of a health educational and exercise program for older adults with osteoarthritis for the hip or knee. The Journal of Rheumatology. 2000;**27**(8):1947-1954

[99] Juhakoski R, Tenhonen S, Malmivaara A, et al. A pragmatic randomized controlled study of the effectiveness and cost consequences of exercise therapy in hip osteoarthritis. Clinical Rehabilitation. 2011;**25**(4):370-383

[100] Krauss I, Steinhilber B, Haupt G, et al. Exercise therapy in hip osteoarthritis—A randomized controlled trial. Deutsches Arzteblatt International. 2014;**111**(35-36): 592-599

[101] Carlson NL. A pilot study on the effects of strength and aerobic coniditioning in patients with hip osteoarthritis. Osteoarthritis and Cartilage. 2011;**S53**:256

[102] Tak E, Staats P, Van Hespen A, et al. The effects of an exercise program for older adults with osteoarthritis of the hip. The Journal of Rheumatology. 2005;**32**(6):1106-1113

[103] Teirlinck CH, Luijsterburg PA, Dekker J, et al. Effectiveness of exercise therapy added to general practitioner care in patients with hip osteoarthritis: A pragmatic randomized controlled trial. Osteoarthritis and Cartilage. 2016;**24**(1):82-90

[104] Loureiro A, Mills PM, Barrett RS. Muscle weakness in hip osteoarthritis: A systematic review. Arthritis Care & Research (Hoboken). 2013;**65**(3):340-352

[105] Marks R. Comorbid depression and anxiety impact hip osteoarthritis disability. Disability and Health Journal. 2009;**2**(1):27-35

[106] van Dijk GM, Veenhof C, Schellevis F, et al. Comorbidity, limitations in activities and pain in patients with osteoarthritis of the hip or knee. BMC Musculoskeletal Disorders. 2008;**9**:95

[107] Bieler T, Siersma V, Magnusson SP, et al. In hip osteoarthritis, Nordic walking is superior to strength

training and home-based exercise for improving function. Scandinavian Journal of Medicine & Science in Sports. 2017;**27**(8):873-886

[108] Cibulka MT, Bloom NJ, Enseki KR, et al. Hip pain and mobility deficits-hip osteoarthritis: Revision 2017. The Journal of Orthopaedic and Sports Physical Therapy. 2017;**47**(6):A1-A37

[109] Messier SP, Callahan LF, Golightly YM, et al. OARSI clinical trials recommendations: Design and conduct of clinical trials of lifestyle diet and exercise interventions for osteoarthritis. Osteoarthritis and Cartilage. 2015;**23**(5):787-797

[110] Lane NE, Hochberg MC, Nevitt MC, et al. OARSI clinical trials recommendations: Design and conduct of clinical trials for hip osteoarthritis. Osteoarthritis and Cartilage. 2015;**23**(5):761-771

[111] McAlindon TE, Bannuru RR, Sullivan MC, et al. OARSI guidelines for the non-surgical management of knee osteoarthritis. Osteoarthritis and Cartilage. 2014;**22**(3):363-388

[112] World Health Organization. International Classification of Functioning, Disability, and Health. Geneva, Switzerland: ICF; 2001

[113] Hefford C, Abbott JH, Baxter GD, et al. Outcome measurement in clinical practice: Practical and theoretical issues for health related quality of life (HRQOL) questionnaires. Physical Therapy Reviews. 2011;**16**(3):155-167

[114] Stratford PW, Kennedy DM, Woodhouse LJ. Performance measures provide assessments of pain and function in people with advanced osteoarthritis of the hip or knee. Physical Therapy. 2006;**86**(11):1489-1496

[115] Abbott JH, Schmitt J. Minimum important differences for the patient-specific functional scale, 4 region-specific outcome measures, and the numeric pain rating scale. The Journal of Orthopaedic and Sports Physical Therapy. 2014;**44**(8):560-564

[116] Tubach F, Ravaud P, Baron G, et al. Evaluation of clinically relevant changes in patient reported outcomes in knee and hip osteoarthritis: The minimal clinically important improvement. Annals of the Rheumatic Diseases. 2005;**64**(1):29-33

[117] Horn KK, Jennings S, Richardson G, et al. The patient-specific functional scale: Psychometrics, clinimetrics, and application as a clinical outcome measure. The Journal of Orthopaedic and Sports Physical Therapy. 2012;**42**(1):30-42

[118] Kamper SJ, Maher CG, Mackay G. Global rating of change scales: A review of strengths and weaknesses and considerations for design. The Journal of Manual & Manipulative Therapy. 2009;**17**(3):163-170

[119] ten Klooster PM, Drossaers-Bakker KW, Taal E, et al. Patient-perceived satisfactory improvement (PPSI): Interpreting meaningful change in pain from the patient's perspective. Pain. 2006;**121**(1-2):151-157

[120] McHorney CA, Ware JE Jr, Raczek AE. The MOS 36-Item Short-form Health Survey (SF 36): II. Psychometric and clinical tests of validity in measuring physical and mental health constructs. Medical Care. 1993;**31**(3):247-263

[121] EuroQol Group. EuroQol—A new facility for the measurement of health-related quality of life. Health Policy (Amsterdam, Netherlands). 1990;**16**(3):199-208

[122] Whitfield K, Buchbinder R, Segal L, et al. Parsimonious and efficient assessment of health-related quality of life in osteoarthritis research: Validation of the Assessment of Quality of Life (AQoL) instrument. Health and Quality of Life Outcomes. 2006;**4**:19

[123] Rat A-C, Pouchot J, Coste J, et al. Development and testing of a specific quality-of-life questionnaire for knee and hip osteoarthritis: OAKHQOL (OsteoArthritis of Knee Hip Quality of Life). Joint, Bone, Spine. 2006;**73**(6):697-704

[124] Mohtadi NG, Griffin DR, Pedersen ME, et al. The development and validation of a self-administered quality-of-life outcome measure for young, active patients with symptomatic hip disease: The International Hip Outcome Tool (iHOT-33). Arthroscopy: The Journal of Arthroscopic & Related Surgery: Official Publication of the Arthroscopy Association of North America and the International Arthroscopy Association. 2012;**28**(5):595-605 quiz 6-10.e1

[125] Kemp JL, Collins NJ, Roos EM, et al. Psychometric properties of patient-reported outcome measures for hip arthroscopic surgery. The American Journal of Sports Medicine. 2013;**41**(9):2065-2073

[126] Martin RL, Philippon MJ. Evidence of reliability and responsiveness for the hip outcome score. Arthroscopy: The Journal of Arthroscopic & Related Surgery: Official Publication of the Arthroscopy Association of North America and the International Arthroscopy Association. 2008;**24**(6):676-682

[127] Bellamy N, Carette S, Ford PM, et al. Osteoarthritis antirheumatic drug trials. III. Setting the delta for clinical trials—Results of a consensus development (Delphi) exercise. The Journal of Rheumatology. 1992;**19**(3):451-457

[128] Wright AA, Cook CE, Baxter GD, et al. A comparison of 3 methodological approaches to defining major clinically important improvement of 4 performance measures in patients with hip osteoarthritis. The Journal of Orthopaedic and Sports Physical Therapy. 2011;**41**:319-327

[129] Mellor R, Bennell K, Grimaldi A, et al. Education plus exercise versus corticosteroid injection use versus a wait and see approach on global outcome and pain from gluteal tendinopathy: Prospective, single blinded, randomised clinical trial. BMJ (Clinical Research Ed). 2018;**361**:k1662

[130] Kivlan BR, Martin RL. Functional performance testing of the hip in athletes: A systematic review for reliability and validity. International Journal of Sports Physical Therapy. 2012;**7**(4):402-412

[131] Fearon AM, Ganderton C, Scarvell JM, et al. Development and validation of a VISA tendinopathy questionnaire for greater trochanteric pain syndrome, the VISA-G. Manual Therapy. 2015;**20**(6):805-813

[132] Crossley KM, Zhang WJ, Schache AG, et al. Performance on the single-leg squat task indicates hip abductor muscle function. The American Journal of Sports Medicine. 2011;**39**(4):866-873

[133] Kinzey SJ, Armstrong CW. The reliability of the star-excursion test in assessing dynamic balance. The Journal of Orthopaedic and Sports Physical Therapy. 1998;**27**(5):356-360

[134] Thorborg K, Hölmich P, Christensen R, et al. The Copenhagen Hip and Groin Outcome Score (HAGOS): Development and validation according to the COSMIN checklist.

British Journal of Sports Medicine. 2011;**45**(6):478-491

[135] Sheean AJ, Schmitz MR, Ward CL, et al. Assessment of disability related to femoroacetabular impingement syndrome by use of the patient-reported outcome measure information system (PROMIS) and objective measures of physical performance. The American Journal of Sports Medicine. 2017;**45**(11):2476-2482

[136] Dobson F, Hinman RS, Hall M, et al. Reliability and measurement error of the Osteoarthritis Research Society International (OARSI) recommended performance-based tests of physical function in people with hip and knee osteoarthritis. Osteoarthritis and Cartilage. 2017;**25**(11):1792-1796

[137] Dobson F, Hinman RS, Roos EM, et al. OARSI recommended performance-based tests to assess physical function in people diagnosed with hip or knee osteoarthritis. Osteoarthritis and Cartilage. 2013;**21**(8):1042-1052

[138] Bellamy N, Buchanan WW, Goldsmith CH, et al. Validation study of WOMAC: A health status instrument for measuring clinically important patient relevant outcomes to antirheumatic drug therapy in patients with osteoarthritis of the hip or knee. The Journal of Rheumatology. 1988;**15**(12):1833-1840

[139] Klassbo M, Larsson E, Mannevik E. Hip disability and osteoarthritis outcome score. An extension of the Western Ontario and McMaster Universities Osteoarthritis Index. Scandinavian Journal of Rheumatology. 2003;**32**(1):46-51

Chapter 4

Hip Arthroplasty

Carlos Roberto Galia, Tiango Aguiar Ribeiro, Cristiano Valter Diesel, Marcelo Reuwsaat Guimarães and Fernando Pagnussato

Abstract

Hip replacement is one of the most performed surgical procedures in orthopedic hip surgery. Through this surgery, the patient returns to most of his normal life and a life without pain. The primary indication for a hip arthroplasty remains osteoarthritis (OA). OA is a degenerative disease that affects synovial joints. A successful surgery is always preceded by good planning. The planning in turn takes into account the analysis of the patient and his physical examination and the radiological image. But also, the surgical planning must take into account another important factor, the choice of the surgical approach. In this chapter, the authors script a revision on the history of hip arthroplasty, total hip arthroplasty approaches, implant types, complications associated with hip arthroplasty, outcomes, and perspectives to the future. We wish you a good reading.

Keywords: bone biology, hip arthroplasty, total hip arthroplasty, orthopedic

1. Introduction and history of hip arthroplasty

The hip arthroplasty is considered one of the greatest achievements of modern orthopedics [1, 2]. Through this surgery the patient returns to most of his normal life and a life without pain [3]. The primary indication for a hip arthroplasty remains osteoarthritis (OA). OA is a degenerative disease that affects synovial joints [4]. Because of the rapid recovery and return to most of the activities of daily living, hip arthroplasty was considered one of the few medical procedures with great benefit to the patient as a whole [5], and this surgery was considered the operation of the century by one of the most important medical journals in 2007 [3].

Hip arthroplasty began in Berlin in the late nineteenth century. Themistocles Gluck fashioned heads in ivory to replace the femoral head. This is the first concept of partial hip arthroplasty or hemiarthroplasty prosthesis. Gluck did these experiments in human patients with hip tuberculosis. These experiments demonstrated that the human body is tolerant to foreign bodies [6, 7]. Schmaltz (1817) and White (1821) underwent hip resection arthroplasty for children patients with hip tuberculosis, and they had been successful. This technique was described by Girdlestone in 1943 [8]. Smith-Petersen in Boston (1923) developed studies coating prosthetic glass, bakelite, and synthetic resin [9]. Philip Wiles (1938) [10] in London brought the concept of a femoral head attached to a rod. The first concept of an acetabular reaming was developed, so was born the concept of total hip arthroplasty (THA). Sir John Charnley [11] was the orthopedist who changed the concept of THA. His early experiments with Teflon have failed. But he developed the concepts of low-friction arthroplasty [12] provided by decreasing the friction area due to the reduction in the diameter of the femoral head (22 mm). And, he used the high-molecular-weight polyethylene associated with methyl methacrylate (cement) [13] developed by Leon Wiltse in Los Angeles. These concepts of alliance were the concepts that changed the course of history of THA surgery. Notice that Haboush was the first orthopedic surgeon to use prosthesis with this cement. Muller was another important surgeon who introduced the prosthesis design with a 32-mm-diameter head [9]. But problems related to cementation generate concerns to improve the cementing techniques. But it was not just that, the search for a better cementation techniques grew. Miller [14] developed the low-viscosity cement, Harris [15, 16] describes techniques for improving cementing, and Robin Ling [17] emphasized the pressurization of the cement in the femoral canal. Despite the problems of cementing, orthopedic surgeons sought new fixation techniques. Pioneers in the area Pillar [18, 19] and Galante [20] introduced the concepts of cementless prosthetic components and the bone growth and pressurization (press fit). The hip arthroplasty surgery is still currently growing and developing. There are several new possibilities: articular surfaces of materials with less friction, more resistant materials, and minimally invasive techniques.

In this chapter, the major aspects of THA surgery will be addressed.

2. Total hip arthroplasty approaches

A successful surgery is always preceded by good planning. The planning in turn takes into account the analysis of the patient and his physical examination and the radiological image. But also, the surgical planning must take into account another important factor, the choice of the surgical approach. The lateral, anterior, and posterior are the main approaches to perform hip arthroplasty. The Moore approach, also named posterior approach [21], is the most used surgical approach. The visibility of the surgical field is wide, and the anatomical approach when known by the surgeon becomes fast and easily accessible. Acetabular and femoral reaming becomes easy to perform due to extensive visibility. Even with an extensive visibility, some authors reported an increased incidence of luxation when this approach is compared to the lateral approach. However, other studies have shown that there is no such correlation [22, 23] and these authors attributed the excessive luxation to the incorrect position of the prosthetic components [22, 23]. Another great and important positive point of this surgical approach is that it does not harm the abductor tendons, so it does not cause limping for operated patients. The lower frequency of deep vein thrombosis (DVT) and bleeding is attributed to this surgical access [22–27]. The anterior surgical approach described by Smith-Petersen [28] and Hueter [29] is less used today, but it has gained new and notorious space among hip surgeons, due to its facilities and strengths for not detaching tendons and muscles. In the same way today, this approach is being used in less invasive and less aggressive surgeries, with the so-called mini-open approach. To the anterior approach, appropriate surgical instruments are needed, and the chance for lesion to occur in the femoral cutaneous nerve during surgery is elevated [30]. The last of the three most commonly used approaches is the direct lateral approach or Hardinge [31]. It has been the most used surgical technique. Hardinge approach is useful because it allows easy placement of the components and it is a familiar approach to a large number of surgeons. This feature makes Hardinge one of the most widely used approaches. Some authors attribute to this approach lower luxation rates than the posterior approach of Moore. But its drawback is that it is able to injure the abductor muscles and cause limping in the patient [22–24].

3. Implant types

The choice of the implant type must also be regarded as extremely important to the success of the surgery. Basically, the implants used in hip arthroplasty can be divided into two groups: non-cemented (cementless implants) and cemented. This division is in regard to the different ways of fixation of the implant to the host patient bone. The main characteristic that distinguishes them is the presence or absence of bone cement (polymethyl methacrylate (PMMA)). Alternatively, a hybrid implant may be used, i.e., a component is fixed with PMMA and other not.

The cemented implants wear the interposition of a polymer called PMMA as an interface between the patient's bone and the implant. This form of attachment was designed by Haboush and subsequently disseminated by Charnley in the 1960s [32]. PMMA has a modulus of elasticity very close to the human bone elasticity modulus (elasticity modulus cement +2GPa; elasticity modulus of trabecular bone +0.5–1GPa). This polymer is very resistant to compressive forces but does not have good resistance to tension or shearing forces [33]. The long-term results to cemented implants depend on the quality of the cement mantle both in the acetabulum and in the femur. Initially, the placement of the cement manually, without the use of distal plug in the femoral canal, was used. The cement mixture was done manually, and pressurization into the canal was performed digitally. This technique was first called as the generation cementing technique. The retrograde filling of the femoral canal with the aid of cement pistols was later developed. They began to use femoral canal plug or plug restrictors, which aims to create a distal barrier to the stem that prevents the passage of cement and favors the pressurization and interdigitation of PMMA in the trabecular bone [34]. These advances represent the second generation of cementation. In the third generation, special techniques were introduced to the cement mixture (vacuum mixing or mixture in centrifuge). However, these special techniques for cement mixing are controversial and do not seem to improve the mechanical properties of PMMA [35]. One of the parameters often used to define an appropriate cementation is the presence of a uniform cement mantle, that is, with no bubbles or lines of radiolucency between the cement and the bone [36]. The thickness of the PMMA mantle is another parameter to define appropriate cementation. In this case, a thickness of 2 mm of the mantle between the femoral stem and the bone is considered adequate [36]. In the acetabulum, the mantle must have a thickness of 3 mm [37]. This trivial standard of cementation has the contrast of the controversial "French paradox," a way of cementation in which the femoral canal is filled with the largest possible stem by using the PMMA to fill the remaining spaces, sometimes getting fine and nonuniform mantels [38]. Other aspects in cemented implants to be observed carefully are:

1. Design—Cemented femoral stems can be classified as simple wedge, double wedge, or triple wedge according to the geometry of the implant. Typical representatives of these subcategories are the stems of Charnley, Exeter, and C-stem, respectively [39]. Although the triple-wedge stems have lower stress in the cement mantle [40], a higher posterior rotation of this implant model is reported [41]. The clinical implications of these findings in the triple-wedge stem are not yet known, and yet this stem type has not demonstrated superiority over other designs [42]. Currently, the stems in double wedge are most often used.

2. The covering of the implant—Traditionally, the best results are obtained with polished implants, i.e., smooth rods. There are femoral stems with rough surface, but these implants are not widely accepted, and its long-term results are not well established in large series [43].

3. The implant material—Usually, the implants are made of chrome-cobalt alloys or stainless steel. Titanium implants were tested; however, the results were very short compared to the traditional metal alloy [44].

The cementless implant aims to obtain a biological fixation between the implant and the host bone. Summarized there is the expectation of bone growth to the porosity of the implant and thus its final attachment to the bone. Unlike cemented implants, the presence of porosity is an indispensable requisite for fixation. There is the use of PMMA in this technique of placing the uncemented prosthesis. The implants do not depend on the cemented macrolocking (primary fixation) and microlocking (secondary fixation). Macrolocking must occur upon insertion of the implant, being obtained by an intimate fit of the implant to the bone. Microlocking is due to the bone ingrowth, i.e., the formation of bony bridges between the host bone and the pores of the implant [45, 46]. Ultimately, this is the factor that determines the longevity and success of a cementless implant. Macrolocking or primary locking can be obtained by various techniques, dependent or not in changes in the design of the implant, such as screw fixing, flaps, or grooves. Currently, the most common technique in primary stabilization is the press fit. This type of stabilization requires the placement of the prosthesis in an undersized cavity. In cementless acetabular beyond the press fit, screws may also be used as an aid to the primary fixation; however, with a suitable press fit, screws can even be dispensed [46–48]. To bone ingrowth occur, macrolocking must produce sufficient stability in order to avoid micromotion. When micromotion occurs, even if slight, it can delay or prevent the formation of bone tissue onto the implant, thus favoring the formation of fibrous tissue [46–49]. For microlocking, porosities are indispensable in the implant surface. Thus, it becomes extremely important different characteristics of the pores, as its size, its geometry, and its interconnection. Studies show that the size of the pores should be between 100 and 400 μm. Pores smaller than 50 μm or greater than 500 μm facilitate the growth of fibrous tissue rather than bone tissue [49]. The pores may have different geometries. There are three traditional types of porosity: the plasma-sprayed coating, the sintered sphere coating, and the fiber mesh coating [49]. In recent years, derived surfaces of trabecular metal porous coating has proven promising in the coverage or in the production of cementless implant, but results with longer follow-up are still waited. It is estimated that the percentage porosity is greater for the fiber mesh coating—between 40 and 50%—and the porous trabecular metal coating—between 75 and 80% [50]. The interconnection between the pores also plays an essential role in bone coupling force to the implant. If it is higher, the interconnection between the pores is resulting in major coupling force between the bone bridges and the prosthesis. Theoretically, the form of the manufacturing fiber mesh coating and the trabecular metal coating allows for a better interconnection between the pores compared to the plasma-sprayed coating and the sphere coating [47].

Another type of arthroplasty are considered hybrid. In this type of prosthesis, one of the implants is cemented and the other does not. It was called hybrid arthroplasty prosthesis in the acetabulum, which is not a cemented and cementless femoral stem. The reverse, i.e., cemented and cementless acetabular rod, was called reverse hybrid arthroplasty.

With regard loading surfaces, tribology has also shown its importance in modern times and has contributed to the THA surgery that increased its longevity. The tribological pair most widely used and studied is the metal-polyethylene. Other tribological pairs are also used: ceramic-polyethylene, metal–metal, and ceramic–ceramic; these last two tribological pairs are also called hard on hard. Currently, there is a trend in replacing the ultrahigh-molecular-weight polyethylene

(UHMWPE) by highly cross-linked polyethylene (XLPE). The XLPE result of a series of interventions during its production seeks to change the connections between the molecules, resulting in a harder and wear-resistant material [51]. It is estimated that 0.04 mm/year is the linear wear rate compared to the XLPE 0:22 mm/year UHMWPE [52, 53]. All new tribological pairs presented as benefit a less volumetric wear, a fact that in theory could be beneficial for the longevity of the arthroplasty. There are, however, some peculiarities in these pairs. The metal–metal surface has an extremely low volumetric wear; however, it is given to metal–metal surface to release chromium and cobalt ions, which can be adsorbed and present local and systemic complications [54]. Among the local complications, pseudotumor formation is the major problem [55]. Systemic effects include neurological and cardiac damage [56]. There are also carcinogenic potential of systemic release of chromium and cobalt, although the exact impact of this exposure is not well known [57]. These systemic effects led to a metal–metal contraindicated in patients with allergies to metals and, in particular, women of childbearing age [58]. The ceramic–ceramic tribological pair has greater resistance to volumetric wear than metal–metal surface. This combination is particularly suitable for very young patients with high activity level and has no contraindication for women of childbearing age. The disadvantages of ceramic–ceramic are fracture risk and the risk of producing noise (squeaking) during hip movement and the stripe wear. The risk of squeaking is multifactorial; the main factors are the malposition of the components, the implant design, and the type of material used in manufacturing, though not always the trigger is recognized [59, 60]. The risk of ceramic fracture is currently between 0.004 and 0.010% being associated with the wrong positioning of the components (acetabular or femoral head) [61]. The stripe wear can occur when there is decreased contact area between the femoral head and acetabular surface, which can arise during swing phase of gait occurs or when the impingement of the trunnion on the acetabular rim and ball leaves right from the socket. The stripe wear is of concern due to the large volumetric wear it can cause. Individuals with tissue hyperlaxity or excellent range of motion (ROM) and those who require placing the hip through the extreme ROM are prone to impingement and consequent stripe wear [62]. The cross-linked polyethylene-ceramic surface adds the benefits of not releasing metal ions, no risk of squeaking besides presenting a very low volumetric wear, however higher than that of the hard-on-hard surfaces. As the head of ceramic is used, there is a minimal risk of fracture of the component. Perhaps, it represents a suitable alternative for young patients and factors that may complicate the use of other types of tribological pairs.

The proper choice of the type of implant, whether cemented or not, and the different tribological pairs should take into account the theoretical knowledge of the design features, materials, and long-term outcomes beyond the patient characteristics and the surgeon's experience.

4. Complications

Complications associated with hip arthroplasty can vary among groups of patients—age, gender, bone quality, and comorbid. For classification purposes it can be divided by time: acute complications, as in intraoperative and early adverse events—generally within 30–90 days, and late postoperative complications that can be divided in short-term and long-term complications. The most common major complications include mortality, infection, dislocation, revision, and thromboembolic events and will be the center of discussion in this section [63].

4.1 Mortality

The indications for arthroplasty have been expanded during recent years. More patients, both younger and old, are operated now, and, in that case, the older group runs a particularly greater natural risk of serious complications. That implicates that higher-risk patients undergo operation than anteriorly. In most recent registries, the short-term mortality rate (90-day mortality) in all patients who undergo hip arthroplasty has an average value of 6.9% [64]. In that period, the dominant causes seem to be cardiac, cerebrovascular, or thromboembolic illnesses. Mortality at 90 days postoperatively in the US Medicare population has been reported as 1% for primary total hip arthroplasty [63]. That shows that mortality can vary significantly, especially when specific groups are studied. In other registries when we divided the mortality rate of partial primary hip replacement—usually used in elderly patients with fractures, we find a rate of 21.53 per 100 person-years. Otherwise, the total primary hip replacement has a rate of 2.54 per 100 person-years [65].

4.2 Thromboembolism

Thromboembolism is a potentially catastrophic complication faced by all patients who undergo elective hip arthroplasty. During the 90 days following primary arthroplasty surgery, hospitalization due to symptomatic deep vein thrombosis occurs in 0.7%, while hospitalization due to pulmonary embolism occurs in 0.3% [66]. In early reports prior of routine prophylaxis, venous thrombosis occurred as high as 50% of times in patients after total hip replacement [67]. In 2001, the sixth conference held by the American College of Chest Physicians came to the conclusion that all patients undergoing total joint replacement needed to be placed in the highest-risk category for DVT [68]. Today, there are guidelines from different medical areas with the intent to patronize the use of drugs and to give information about the management of thromboembolic disease. Despite all the attempts to validate and embrace the use of these guidelines, the ideal method of thromboembolic events prophylaxis remains controversial.

The general concern for total joint replacement surgeons, about these publications considered as high-level recommendations (1A), was the promotion of aggressive treatment for all patients, regardless of their risk profile. In 2011 and 2012, reports from the FDA appointed that anticoagulants were the leading drug risk to patients and complications like bleeding, drainage, and wound complications were the critical counterpoint for routine aggressive prophylaxis [69].

Today, there is no current evidence whether factors other than a history of previous venous thromboembolism increase the risk of venous thromboembolism in patients undergoing elective hip arthroplasty [70]. There are many other factors that were appointed to increase risk, like, obesity, or advanced age, but there's no real evidence to support. There is a consensus that any other factor that can cause decrease of mobility can be a risk factor, the same way for hemostatic abnormalities that can cause hypercoagulable states. There are no image exams or laboratory markers that can indicate a greater risk for thromboembolism. Today, there is strong evidence against the routine use of ultrasound for the screening of patients after hip arthroplasty for DVT. Is important to bear in mind that, at least 50% of patients, diagnose is not clinically apparent.

The diagnosis of DVT is based in clinical findings, usually pain and tenderness in the calf or thigh, erythema, and swelling, most of the times unilateral. Venography still stands as the "gold standard" for confirmation of DVT, but the duplex ultrasound seems to be a low-cost, minimal morbidity, good sensitivity option, besides the risk of anaphylactic reaction to contrast and low chances of inducing DVT that venography carries. Pulmonary embolism can curse with chest pain, breathlessness, and rapid pulse, and it's a cause of sudden death. The diagnosis can be confirmed by pulmonary angiography.

The best method of prophylaxis still is not clear. There is evidence to suggest that pharmacological agents and/or mechanical compression devices reduce DVT rates in patients undergoing elective knee or hip arthroplasty. The results of analyses in recent studies did not consistently suggest that any one strategy is preferable to another. The most commonly used agents are low-molecular-weight heparin (LMWH), aspirin, direct factor Xa inhibitors ("xabans"), and warfarin. Devices of intermittent compression seem to be effective especially in distal emboli. There's no consensus either for the time that prophylaxis is maintained. It varies for at least 10 days as far as 35 days after surgery, depending on the patient and the drug. There has been a tendency to return the use of aspirin after hospital discharge [71].

It is a consensus, even when there's no evidence to support, that patients undergoing elective hip or knee arthroplasty, and who also have a known bleeding disorder (e.g., hemophilia) and/or active liver disease, use a less aggressive treatment with mechanical compressive devices for preventing venous thromboembolism.

Early mobilization still is a low-cost, minimal risk to the patient and consistent method with the current practice. Mobilization as soon as possible following hip arthroplasty addresses the stasis limb of Virchow's triad (hypercoagulability, endothelial injury, and stasis) promoting the regional blood flow and diminishing the risk for formation of clots.

4.3 Dislocation

Dislocation is one of the most feared complications after THA. Probably, it is one of the most common indications for revision surgery. An incidence from 1 to 3% of dislocation after THA has been reported [72]. Risk factors include the type of surgical approach, previous surgery, obesity, fracture of proximal femur, malpositioning of components, impingement, insufficient abductor muscle, femoral component head sizes, and others. Many studies tried to isolated these causes, but there's not much medical evidence to support, and the most common conclusion is that retrospective randomized trials examining dislocation rates and other clinical parameters are needed [73]. Clinical finding include pain, shortening, and internal or external rotation of the limb.

Factors like age, height, or race are seen to be associated with bias with at least one technical-related factor when the disclosure is dislocation. However, in many series, dislocation occurred in women more often than men.

The most used surgical approaches for THA are the posterior and direct lateral approaches. The posterior approach is considered to be easy to perform; however, increased rates of dislocation have been reported. The direct lateral approach was related to an increased risk of limp. Studies indicate that soft tissue repair reduces the relative risk of dislocation using the posterior approach and that the dislocation rate for these approaches becomes similar. It has been advocated that bigger head sizes increase instability and have greater ROM [22, 74, 75].

The vast majority of dislocations occur within 3 months of surgery. These early dislocation (<6 months) presents higher chance of success with nonoperative treatment. Late complications, after 5 years in general, are more challenging to treat because of the many factors that can be attributed to these cases [72]. The combination of muscular weakness and malposition implants is seen to be the worst scenario for hip stability.

Besides all the discussion about head sizes and different approaches, the single, most effective way of preventing dislocation still is education of the patients and the people who assist them. They should be aware that which extreme movements and which specific position are most likely to cause dislocation, and the ways of avoid them without lose their independence. It's important that the patient is able to repeat and understand the instructions for precaution before hospital discharge and has reinforced these directions at follow-up routine.

The surgical options for treatment are as many as the causes for the dislocation can be. Change of components for longer and bigger heads, liner exchange, and elevated rim could be successful sometimes; otherwise, component revision, soft tissue reconstruction, or even constrained liner may be needed. Identifying the causes of instability after THA is essential for the correct approach and satisfactory outcome.

4.4 Nerve and vascular injuries

Nerve and vascular injuries are very uncommon complications in primary total hip replacement but can be the most distressing ones. With an incidence between 0.8 and 3.5% for nerve injuries, the most common nerve damage followed by femoral nerve has been the sciatic nerve palsy [76]. These numbers can be altered when you observe a specific kind of approach, as with the anterior direct approach, that can present with up to 15% of lateral femoral cutaneous nerve palsy in some reports [77].

Several risk factors were identified for nerve injuries, including previous surgery, revision procedures, type of approach, and excessive leg extension. However, no correlation between the amount of lengthening and nerve palsy in total arthroplasties performed for dysplasia of the hip has been reported [78]. Previous surgery or revisions were correlated with technically difficult in the surgical exposure, anatomical abnormalities, and injudicious retraction. In order to diagnose nerve palsy after orthopedic surgery, an electromyogram can be of use to assess the extent and prognosis. According to the literature, partial recovery can be expected in 70–80% of cases. Latest reports appoint only 50% of full recovery after common peroneal nerve palsy following total hip arthroplasty with the mean time of 12–18 mouths depending on the severity of lesion. Other studies showed improvement beyond the limit of 2 years and independent of the nerve affected. Obesity was appointed as a factor that adversely influenced the nerve recovery [79, 80].

Vascular injury in primary hip arthroplasty is rare and most frequently associated with the use of screws for fixation of structural grafts, acetabular components, and protrusio rings or cages. The individual risk is determined by multiple factors depending on the surgeon's skills, the number of previous surgeries, and the approach itself. The acetabular quadrant system as described by Wasielewski et al. is a useful tool to understand the neurovascular anatomy of the hip, to detect the safe zone, and subsequently prevents complications that can pose as a threat to the limb and the patient [81].

4.5 Fractures

The most common are those who affect the femur and are classified by the local of the fracture, the fixation of implant, and the bone stock of the femur. Can also be dived by time, as intraoperative and postoperative fractures, the most common being the intraoperative fractures of the femur with an uncemented steam.

There are moments during the procedure that the fracture is most likely to occur. One of the critical stages seems to be while attempting to dislocate the hip, especially in fragile bones of elderly patients and rheumatoid arthritis patients. During the stage of broaching or during the insertion of the implant, cortical defects and proximal deformities can elicit a fracture of the diaphysis. Acetabular fractures are much more uncommon also because often they are not recognized. The key moment is seen to be, with press-fit components, during the impaction of an underreamed acetabulum.

The Vancouver classification of periprosthetic femoral fractures became known for postoperative fractures and was modified to include this intraoperative ones (**Table 1**).

The treatment can be initiated by taking preventive actions: the anticipation of anatomical challenges in preoperative planning and templating; the choice of implants, by the use of moderate rotational force and with wider approaches; and the liberation of soft tissues that might be restraining to the adequate exposure. Patients with osteoporotic bone, neuromuscular disorders, and previous hip surgery should be of higher concern. The use of fluoroscopy is an important tool to identify these fractures when suspected. Each type of fracture needs a specific treatment. In a review by Misur et al. [83], they summarize recommendations for the treatment of periprosthetic fractures of the femur with grading of published evidence supporting each recommendation (**Table 2**). The need for adjunctive fixation should be assessed, extended approach for the correct assessment is often needed, and the result needs to present a stable construction. Clear orientation for the patient and family about weight-bearing and healing process of the fracture is essential for good results.

4.6 Infection

Periprosthetic joint infection remains a challenge for the orthopedic surgeons. It represents a risk for disastrous and painful consequences for the patients, especially for those submitted to elective primary joint replacement. The incidence reports approximately 1% of infection after THA. Great effort is applied to identify risk factors, minimize, and prevent these complications in a systematic way. Currently, recommendations are based in large, multicenter studies, but still high-level evidence for these practices are few, and many are based on little to none scientific

	Vancouver A		Vancouver B		Vancouver C	
	AG	AL	B1	B2	B3	C
Prosthetic fixation	Stable	Stable	Stable	Loose	Loose	Stable
Bone quality	Good	Good	Good	Good	Poor	Good

Table 1.
Vancouver classification resume [82].

Type AG	Nonoperative treatment if nondisplaced; open reduction and internal fixation if displaced fracture in active patient
Type AL	Nonoperative treatment unless implant stability compromised
Type B1	Fixation with minimally invasive lateral locking plate; addition of allograft strut if bone stock compromised
Type B2	Revision with extensively coated tapered fluted stem (modular or nonmodular)
Type B3	Revision with extensively coated tapered fluted stem (modular or nonmodular); if bone stock grossly compromised, use allograft-prosthesis composite with megaprosthesis reserved for salvage procedures and elderly patients
Type C	Fixation with minimally invasive lateral locking plate

Adapted from [84].

Table 2.
Treatment of periprosthetic fractures of the femur after total hip arthroplasty.

foundation whatsoever. In 2014, the Proceedings of the International Consensus Meeting on Periprosthetic Joint Infection in the attempt to unify the current knowledge and practice was published.

Risk factors were divided as significant and potential risks for development of surgical site infection (SSI) or periprosthetic joint infection (PJI) after elective total joint arthroplasty (TJA). In the first category, 99% of the delegates consensus that active infection of the arthritic joint (septic arthritis), presence of septicemia, and/or presence of active local cutaneous, subcutaneous, or deep tissue infection are all significant risk factors predisposing patients to and are contraindication to undertaking elective TJA. Ninety-four percent agree that history of the previous surgery, poorly controlled diabetes mellitus (glucose > 200 mg/L or HbA1C > 7%), malnutrition, morbid obesity (BMI > 40 Kg/m^2), active liver disease, chronic renal disease, excessive smoking (>1 pack per day), excessive alcohol consumption (>40 units per week), intravenous drug abuse, recent hospitalization, extended stay in a rehabilitation facility, male gender, diagnosis of posttraumatic arthritis, inflammatory arthropathy, prior surgical procedure in the affected joint, and severe immunodeficiency are potential risk factors for development of SSI or PJI [85].

Active infection in periodontal disease, methicillin-resistant *Staphylococcus aureus* (MRSA), and methicillin-sensitive *Staphylococcus aureus* (MSSA) colonization were appointed as factors that can contribute to development of the infection, as well as urinary tract infection (UTI); however, there's no medical evidence to support screening for these patients. Nevertheless, patients with a known history of recurrent urinary infection or for those with evidence of ongoing urinary symptoms suspicious for infection should receive special attention.

Antibiotic prophylaxis is, in general, the most important factor to reduce the chances of contaminating microorganisms to establish during the procedure exposure. For that it's important that, by the time of the incision, there is adequate tissue concentration of the drug. Most of the guidelines recommend that prophylactic antibiotics be completely infused within 1 hour before the surgical incision. A first- or second-generation cephalosporin is normally administered for routine perioperative surgical prophylaxis, mostly because of its broad spectrum of action, cost-effectiveness, and the need to preserve newer and more expensive therapies for drug-resistant microorganisms. Additionally, they have excellent distribution profiles in the bone, synovium, muscle, and hematomas. Patients who weigh more than 80 kg should receive double the amount of cefazolin usually used. The efficacy of 1 day of cefuroxime vs. 3 days of cefazolin on postoperative wound infections was tested and found to have no statistically significant difference between the two regimens [86]. An additional dose of antibiotic should be administered intraoperatively after two half-lives of the prophylactic agent or after important blood loss. The choice of antibiotics for patients with pre-existing prostheses such as heart valves is the same as that for routine elective arthroplasty.

If infection is suspected, it's important to understand in what moment of the disease the patient presents himself because time is a relevant factor in approaching these complications and might influence in the treatment options. There are many classifications; in general, they are divided as follows: (1) early postoperative infection that can vary between 3 and 6 weeks onset within the time of the surgery, depending on the author; (2) late chronic infection after these periods and with an insidious presentation of symptoms; and (3) acute hematogenous infection, defined by the onset after these 3 to 6 weeks in a previously well-functioning prosthesis, probably by a distant source of infection.

The diagnosis still is in debate; the consensus is defined as PJI as follows:

- Two positive periprosthetic cultures with phenotypically identical organisms
- A sinus tract communicating with the joint
- Having three of the following minor criteria:
- Elevated serum C-reactive protein (CRP) and erythrocyte sedimentation rate (ESR)
- Elevated synovial fluid white blood cell (WBC) count OR ++change on leukocyte esterase test strip
- Elevated synovial fluid polymorphonuclear neutrophil percentage (PMN%)
- Positive histological analysis of periprosthetic tissue
- A single positive culture

The AAOS's algorithm (**Figure 1**) was adapted to be applied to patients who present with a painful or failed arthroplasty.

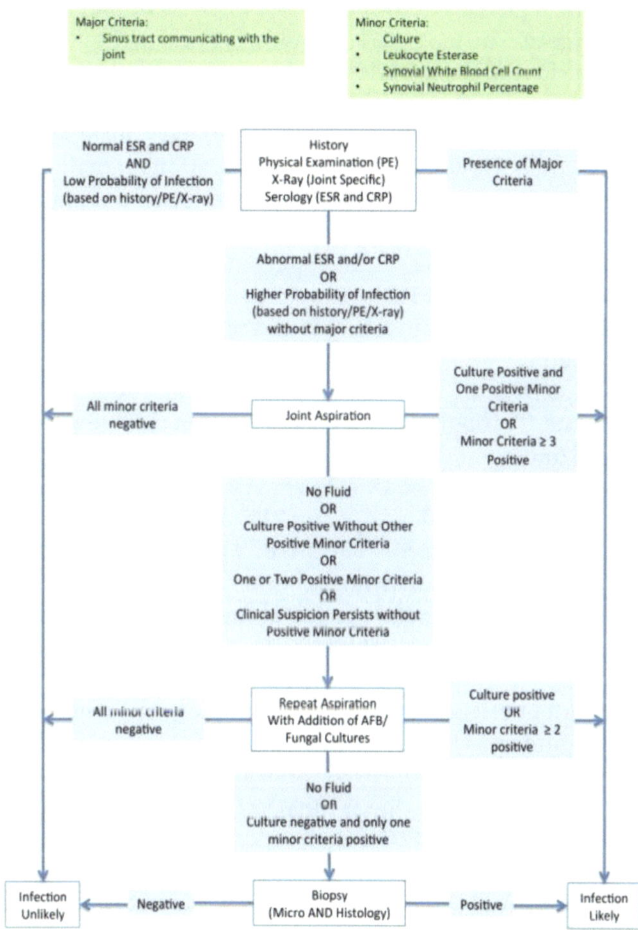

Figure 1.
The AAOS's algorithm for treatment to patients with a painful or failed arthroplasty [85].

The major discussion nowadays among joint replacement hip surgeons is whether to perform a one-stage or two-stage revision in patients with diagnosis of infection. Patients with early postoperative infection apparently have strong chances of cure when an open debridement and change of mobile parts are realized as an early aggressive intervention [87].

Both procedures have the same intent: identification of the organisms; eradication of the foci; physical removal of any organism, tissue, or components that might have been exposed; appropriated treatment with antibiotics; and safe reconstruction of the joint in a healthy environment.

The bone cement loaded with antibiotics has been the main weapon in the one-stage enthusiasts, as the spacers have been for those who advocate four two-stage revisions. The selection of patients has been seen to have an important role in that decision; the tendency has been the single-stage revision. With more studies published each year showing similar outcomes for both types of procedures, the social and economic advantages of one operation, like shorter hospitalization, early return to activities, and higher satisfaction rates, give the one-stage revision an increasing role in the treatment of joint infection.

5. Outcomes

The focus of THA registries traditionally has been on implant longevity and rates of revision surgery. The landmark of failure of the implant and the necessity of revision still are considered the best definition of clinical failure as well. Otherwise, the choice of parameters for the definition of failure, clinical or radiographic, could be troublesome. Short-term mortality rate (90 days postoperative) also has been used as an outcome. However, the latest publications signalize an important change in the outcome reports. Since pain, impaired joint function, and quality of life related to hip disease are the main indications for THA, thus to include this patient-related information in the results reported after primary hip replacement. The patient-reported outcome (PRO) includes pain relief, joint function, and other health-related quality-of-life improvements and represents an important aspect of hip arthroplasty results.

National joint registries are the most reliable and most quoted references when the subject is outcome. Through them it's been possible to have a greater view and more profound understanding of why arthroplasties fail. For example, in the Norwegian report of 2002, 9.2% of 17,323 primary Charnley hip prosthesis implants were revised after 10 years of follow-up, and 71% of the failures involved aseptic loosening of the femoral component. The use of a specific type of cements was appointed as an important and highly significant probable cause in this percentage [88]. Another example was the metal-on-metal surface and the early complications reported in many registries. For that manner, reports became an essential tool to orthopedic surgeons to understand the impact of all these variables—implant design, material, patient selection, surgical techniques, and others—and how they are influencing the outcomes in their clinical practice.

In general the most common causes for revision are the same in every other registry or study published. Sometimes, the percentages can vary depending on the population studied. In the 2012 Swedish reports, for example, aseptic loosening including osteolysis was the most common cause for revision (28%), followed by dislocation (26%), infection (22%), and periprosthetic fracture (13%) [89].

One of the major areas of discussion has been cemented versus cementless implants and how they can influence in the outcome. An increasing use of uncemented implants in the last 10 to 15 years has been reported. Over the same time period, there was a corresponding reduction in the use of cemented ones. The National Joint Registry for England, Wales, Northern Ireland and the Isle of Man of 2014 reports that in 2003 cemented hip replacement was used in 60.5% in comparison to 33.2% in 2013. Otherwise, cementless increased from 16.8% in 2003 to 42.5% in 2013 [90]. The "new trend" defenses of uncemented implants are that it is faster surgically, avoids the third-body debris, and creates a biological interface of bone ingrown in the implant (and with that less rate of loosening) and less chances of embolic events that can occur during cementation. The cement users appoint that there are less fractures, intra- and postoperatively, less dislocation and leg length discrepancies, and less thigh pain report after surgery, and, mainly, there is registry data of better outcome in patients older than 75 years [91].

All these qualities or failures on both implants are, in fact, correct. Cemented hip arthroplasties have been reported to be better in many nation registries, especially in older patients [92, 93]. Otherwise, specific centers across the globe reported up to 99% of cementless steam survival after 12–26 years of follow-up [94, 95]. There are reports of the accuracy during cup position, and cemented cups seem to have better position than uncemented cups that have the tendency to deviate from their original place [96]. The incidence of periprosthetic femoral fractures is becoming more common, and that could be attributed to the larger use of uncemented implants. Thigh pain is most common with uncemented femoral steams, but in a great way, this can be attributed to the design of the implant that was used. The major issue in using cemented implants still is the technique and its reproducibility. Perfect cementing technique is essential to achieve all these excellent results. Pulsatile jet-lavage to clean the cancellous bone and allow the cement to have good interdigitat ing as well as good pressurization and homogenous cement mantle is appointed as prerequisite to reach adequate cementation [97].

Other important aspect of failure in hip arthroplasty has been between the implants that are used in partial arthroplasties. In the Australian report of 2014, in patients under the age of 75 years old after the neck of the femur fracture, the revision rate after 10 years for primary unipolar monoblock and unipolar modular hip replacement was the same (16.1%). To the same group of patients, the bipolar presents a 9% rate of revision in the same period of 10 years [93].

In primary hip replacement for osteoartrite (OA), nation registry reports are similar, in an overall of 5–6% rate of revision in 10 years for all ages. When divided by the type, the British reports 3.2% for all cemented, 7.68% to all cementless implants, and a total of 3.95% for hybrids. The Australian reports 6, 5.4, and 4.8%, respectively. When divided by age and gender, younger females are in greater risk of revision in 10 years. Inversion occurs when the primary replacement is made around 65 years of age in men, showing a slightly higher incidence of revision than women after 10 years [90, 93].

A lot of attention is given to the type of bearing nowadays. The most recent surfaces like ceramics, highly cross-linked polyethylene, and their combination with metal generate a lot of discussion in what would be the ideal, more durable surface, and for whom it should be use. Keeping aside the costs and a few laboratory assays, there is no real evidence in favor or against any of these, except for the metal-on-metal combination that has inferior outcomes in almost all the comparative published. In the 2014 Australian report, ceramic combined with ceramic and highly cross-linked polyethylene had similar 10-year rates, 4.7 and 4.5%, respectively. The lower revision rate was metal on highly cross-linked polyethylene with 4.3% in 1 years. Any of these combinations, when associated with an exchangeable femoral neck, showed two times higher rate of failure in that same period of time [93]. In the British reports, hybrid assembly with ceramic on polyethylene showed the outcome with 2.19% in 10 years [90].

The material that steams are made also has an influence in the outcomes as well as femoral head sizes. Pure titanium seems to have lower revision rates than titanium and cobalt-chrome in the steam/neck material. Head sizes of 32 mm have a lower rate of revision than head sizes of 28 mm or less. However, there is no difference when head size 32 mm is compared to larger head size. This can probably be attributed to the higher incidence of dislocation that 28 mm or less heads present [93].

It has been advocated that total hip arthroplasty is probably the most successful operative intervention performed by human beings. Still, a constant strive for innovation has a guide progress, especially in the technologic field. Every year more aspects are being reported, and a great volume of information has been gathered. More than never before, more patients, with a wider range of age and comorbidities, are having their hips replaced. The understanding of how this affects their lives and how to meet the changes in the demand and expectations for THA is an essential key to keep improving such celebrated medical procedure.

For this reason, patient-reported outcome measures (PROMs) are becoming increasingly important in the allocation of healthcare resources and the provision of guidelines for optimum care and management [89].The Swedish reports were pioneer in that area and are still improving the way to collect this information and how to process that in numbers. In 2012 reports, patient satisfaction 1 year of THA (2010–2011) varied from 82.8 to 93.4%. They analyzed other variables such as pain relief, health-related quality of life gained, 90-day mortality, coverage, reoperation within 2 years, 5-year implant survival, 10-year implant survival, and set and nationwide standard for comparison with the obtained by institutions. The conclusions highlight the great challenge that it's to organize the structure of information and engage the participants. Important influences were appointed related to anxiety and depression in the predictor of pain, pain relief, and patient satisfaction [98]. There's no doubt that this patient-related information will have an increasing role in the advanced hip arthroplasty.

6. Perspectives to the future

Although hip arthroplasty celebrates over 50 years since its creation, how the procedure has been slow in recent years. The main lines of research thus far developed are concentrated in areas that seek alternatives to metal implants, the use of new biomaterials, as well as the use of computer tools for planning and development of surgery [99].

Several studies involving existing prostheses on the market seek to improve efficiency by reducing the rejection or failure and to find synergy between the contact areas. With this, new surfaces, such as porous, the use of mesh titanium, and the development of metal-polyethylene interaction, are being researched [100, 101].

The area of biomaterials points to major advances. Examples are the use of hydroxyapatite for surface coating, the use of alternative bone graft as humans or bovine lyophilized to assist in cases of bone loss, as well as the development of multidisciplinary techniques for bone regeneration, as in the case of VascuBone Project [102–104].

Among the computer tools for programming and development of surgery, the navigation techniques are the most researched. The main distinguishing feature of this feature is that it provides real-time measurements and precise alignments [105–109].

7. Conclusions

Regardless of the approach, the chosen implant, the THA surgery, is a major evolution of modern medicine and came as a great benefit to patients. Every technique employed should be well studied, and the patient must always be the most benefited from the surgery.

Acknowledgements

The authors would like to thank the Federal University of Rio Grande do Sul (UFRGS), Department of Orthopedics, Tissue Bank Unit, at the Hospital de Clínicas de Porto Alegre (HCPA), Porto Alegre, Rio Grande do Sul (RS), Brazil.

Conflict of interest

We hereby indicate that there is no financial or business interest concerning any author or their immediate family members of the manuscript entitled "Hip Arthroplasty." The submitted manuscript is a study on the history of hip arthroplasty, total hip arthroplasty approaches, implant types, complications associated with hip arthroplasty, outcomes, and perspectives to the future.

We also confirm that no conflict of interest for drugs, devices or prosthesis, or any other materials either biological or synthetic exists in this study if they are not being particularly assessed as part of the investigation.

Moreover, no part of the investigation has been carried out or supported in grant by any related company or entity. None of the authors own stock, acted as a consultant, established contract work, served as an officer or member of the board, or received more than US$ 2000 a year from any related company or entity within the past 2 years.

Each author fulfills the requirements for authorship and publicly and legally responds for the content of the above manuscript, and all authors have read this final version of the paper and are aware of its content and agreed with the submitted version of the manuscript.

We assure that the information above is absolutely accurate.

Notes/thanks/other declarations

The authors would like to thank the Research Group in Hip, Biomaterials and Tissue Bank, Hospital de Clínicas de Porto Alegre, Porto Alegre, Rio Grande do Sul, Brazil, for the opportunity in developing this work.

Nomenclature

OA	osteoarthritis
THA	total hip arthroplasty
DVT	deep vein thrombosis
PMMA	polymethyl methacrylate
Gpa	gigapascal
UHMWPE	ultrahigh-molecular-weight polyethylene
XLPE	highly cross-linked polyethylene
ROM	range of motion
LMWH	low-molecular-weight heparin
SSI	surgical site infection
PJI	periprosthetic joint infection
TJA	total joint arthroplasty
BMI	body mass index
MRSA	methicillin-resistant *Staphylococcus aureus*
MSSA	methicillin-sensitive *Staphylococcus aureus*
UTI	urinary tract infection

CRP	C-reactive protein
ESR	erythrocyte sedimentation rate
WBC	white blood cell
PMN%	polymorphonuclear neutrophil percentage
AAOS	American Academy of Orthopaedic Surgeons
PROs	patient-reported outcome
PROMs	patient-reported outcome measures

Author details

Carlos Roberto Galia[1,2,3,4*], Tiango Aguiar Ribeiro[5,6], Cristiano Valter Diesel[2,3], Marcelo Reuwsaat Guimarães[7] and Fernando Pagnussato[2,4,8,9]

1 Surgery Department, Federal University of Rio Grande do Sul (UFRGS), Porto Alegre, Rio Grande do Sul (RS), Brazil

2 Department of Orthopedics, Hospital de Clínicas de Porto Alegre (HCPA), Porto Alegre, Rio Grande do Sul (RS), Brazil

3 Medicine School of Federal University of Rio Grande do Sul (UFRGS), Porto Alegre, Rio Grande do Sul (RS), Brazil

4 Hospital de Clínicas de Porto Alegre (HCPA), Porto Alegre, Rio Grande do Sul (RS), Brazil

5 Surgery Department, Federal University of Santa Maria (UFSM), Santa Maria, Rio Grande do Sul (RS), Brazil

6 Department of Orthopedics (SOT), University Hospital of Santa Maria (UFSM), Santa Maria, Rio Grande do Sul (RS), Brazil

7 Orthopedic and Traumatologist Surgeon, Hospital de Clínicas de Porto Alegre (HCPA), Porto Alegre, Rio Grande do Sul (RS), Brazil

8 Federal University of Rio Grande do Sul. (UFRGS), Porto Alegre, Rio Grande do Sul (RS), Brazil

9 Tissue Bank, Hospital de Clínicas de Porto Alegre (HCPA), Porto Alegre, Rio Grande do Sul (RS), Brazil

*Address all correspondence to: cgalia@hcpa.ufrgs.br

References

[1] Jones CA et al. Health related quality of life outcomes after total hip and knee arthroplasties in a community based population. The Journal of Rheumatology. 2000;**27**(7):1745-1752

[2] Laupacis A et al. The effect of elective total hip replacement on health-related quality of life. The Journal of Bone and Joint Surgery. 1993;**75**(11):1619-1626

[3] Learmonth DC et al. The operation of the century: Total hip replacement. The Lancet. 2007;**370**(9597):1508-1519

[4] Wood AM et al. A review on the management of hip and knee osteoarthritis. International Journal of Chronic Diseases. 2013;**2013**:10

[5] Della Valle CJ, Rosenberg AG. Primary total hip arthroplasty: Indications and contraindications. In: Callaghan JJ, Rosenberg AG, Rubash HE, editors. The Adult Hip. Philadelphia, USA: Lippincott Williams & Wilkins; 2007. pp. 851-858

[6] Gluck T. Die invaginationsmethode der osteo-und arthroplastik. Berliner Klinische Wochenschrift. 1890;**28**: 732-736, 752-757

[7] Haas J. Neue anwendungsgebiete der lorenz'schen bifurkation (gabelung des oberen femurendes). Zentralblatt für Chirurgie. 1927;**54**:783-785

[8] Schwartsmann CR, Boschin LC. Quadril do adulto. In: Hebert S et al., editors. Ortopedia e Traumatologia: Princípios e Prática. Porto Alegre: Artmed Editora S. A.; 2009. pp. 407-442

[9] Peltier LF. A history of hip surgery. In: Callaghan JJ, Rosenberg AG, Rubash HE, editors. The Adult Hip. Philadelphia, USA: Lippincott Williams & Wilkins; 2007. pp. 3-31

[10] Wiles P. The Surgery of the osteoarthritic hip. The British Journal of Surgery. 1958;**45**:488-497

[11] Waugh W. John Charnley: The Man and the Hip. London: Springer-Verlang; 1990

[12] Charnley J. Total hip replacement by low-friction arthroplasty. Clinical Orthopaedics and Related Research. 1970;**72**:7-21

[13] Charnley J. Anchorage of the femoral head prosthesis to the shaft of the femur. The Journal of Bone and Joint Surgery. 1960;**42-B**:28-30

[14] Miller J. Pressure penetration of low viscosity acrylic cement for improved fixation of arthroplasty components. The Journal of Bone and Joint Surgery. 1982;**64**:619

[15] Harris WH, McCarthy JC Jr, O'Neill DA. Femoral component loosening using contemporary techniques of femoral cement fixation. The Journal of Bone and Joint Surgery. 1982;**64**(7):1063-1067

[16] Harris WH, McCarthy JC Jr, O'Neill DA. Loosening of the femoral component of total hip replacement after plugging the femoral canal. The Hip. 1982:228-238. PMID: 7166501. https://www.ncbi.nlm.nih.gov/pubmed/7166501

[17] Lee AJ, Ling RS, Vangala SS. Some clinically relevant variables affecting the mechanical behaviour of bone cement. Archives of Orthopaedic and Trauma Surgery. 1978;**92**(1):1-18

[18] Bobyn JD et al. Porous surfaced layered prosthetic devices. Journal of Biomedical Engineering. 1975;**10**:126-131

[19] Bobyn JD et al. The optimum pore size for the fixation of porous-surfaced metal implants by the ingrowth of bone.

Clinical Orthopaedics and Related Research. 1980;**150**(150):263-270

[20] Galante J. Total hip replacement. The Orthopedic Clinics of North America. 1971;**2**(1):139-155

[21] Moore AT. Metal hip joint; a new self-locking vitallium prosthesis. Southern Medical Journal. 1952;**45**(11):1015-1019

[22] Kwon MS et al. Does surgical approach affect total hip arthroplasty dislocation rates? Clinical Orthopaedics and Related Research. 2006;**447**:34-38

[23] Macedo CAS et al. Comparação das abordagens ântero-lateral e posterior em artroplastia total primária de quadril. Revista Brasileira de Ortopedia. 1997;**32**(10):777-780

[24] Alencar PGC, Abagge M. Artroplastia total do quadril por via de acesso póstero-lateral. Revista Brasileira de Ortopedia. 1995;**30**:509-513

[25] Gore DR et al. Anterolateral compared to posterior approach in total hip arthroplasty: Differences in component positioning, hip strength, and hip motion. Clinical Orthopaedics and Related Research. 1982;**165**:180-187

[26] Vicente JRN et al. A influência da via de acesso na luxação das artroplastias totais do quadril. Revista Brasileira de Ortopedia. 2009;**44**:507-507

[27] Sikorski JM, Hampson WG, Staddon GE. The natural history and aetiology of deep vein thrombosis after total hip replacement. The Journal of Bone and Joint Surgery. 1981;**63-B**(2):171-177

[28] Matta JM, Shahrdar C, Ferguson T. Single-incision anterior approach for total hip arthroplasty on an orthopaedic table. Clinical Orthopaedics and Related Research. 2005;**441**:115-124

[29] DeWal H, Su E, DiCesare PE. Instability following total hip arthroplasty. American Journal of Orthopedics. 2003;**32**(8):377-382

[30] Paillard P. Hip replacement by a minimal anterior approach. International Orthopaedics. 2007;**31**(Suppl. 1):S13-S15

[31] Hardinge K. The direct lateral approach to the hip. The Journal of Bone and Joint Surgery. 1982;**64**(1):17-19

[32] Charnley J. Arthroplasty of the hip. A new operation. Lancet. 1961;**1**(7187):1129-1132

[33] Webb JC, Spencer RF. The role of polymethylmethacrylate bone cement in modern orthopaedic surgery. The Journal of Bone and Joint Surgery. 2007;**89**:851-857

[34] Rice J et al. Femoral cementing techniques in total hip replacement. International Orthopaedics. 1998;**22**(5):308-311

[35] Geiger MH et al. The clinical significance of vacuum mixing bone cement. Clinical Orthopaedics and Related Research. 2001;**382**:258-266

[36] Chambers IR et al. Radiological features predictive of aseptic loosening in cemented Charnley femoral stems. The Journal of Bone and Joint Surgery. 2001;**83**(6):838-842

[37] Ritter MA et al. Radiological factors influencing femoral and acetabular failure in cemented Charnley total hip arthroplasties. The Journal of Bone and Joint Surgery. 1999;**81**(6):982-986

[38] Langlais F et al. The 'French paradox'. The Journal of Bone and Joint Surgery. 2003;**85**(1):17-20

[39] Jayasuriya RL et al. Effect of sliding-taper compared with composite-beam cemented femoral prosthesis loading regime on proximal femoral bone remodeling: A

randomized clinical trial. The Journal of Bone and Joint Surgery. 2013;**95**(1):19-27

[40] New AM, Taylor M, Wroblewski BM. Effect of hip stem taper on cement stresses. Orthopedics. 2005;**28**(8 Suppl):s857-s862

[41] Sundberg M et al. Movement patterns of the C-stem femoral component: An RSA study of 33 primary total hip arthroplasties followed for two years. The Journal of Bone and Joint Surgery. 2005;**87**(10):1352-1356

[42] Ek ET, Choong PF. Comparison between triple-tapered and double-tapered cemented femoral stems in total hip arthroplasty: A prospective study comparing the C-stem versus the exeter universal early results after 5 years of clinical experience. The Journal of Arthroplasty. 2005;**20**(1):94-100

[43] Verdonschot N, Tanck E, Huiskes R. Effects of prosthesis surface roughness on the failure process of cemented hip implants after stem-cement debonding. Journal of Biomedical Materials Research. 1998;**42**(4):554-559

[44] Noiseux NO et al. Uncemented porous tantalum acetabular components: Early follow-up and failures in 613 primary total hip arthroplasties. The Journal of Arthroplasty. 2014;**29**(3):617-620

[45] Blaha JD, Borus TA. Press-fit femoral components. In: Callaghan JJ, Rosenberg AG, Rubash HE, editors. The Adult Hip. Philadelphia: Lippincott Williams & Wilkins; 2007. pp. 1036-1043

[46] Sporer SM, Paprosky WG. Biologic fixation and bone ingrowth. The Orthopedic Clinics of North America. 2005;**36**(1):105-111, vii

[47] Jasty M, Kienapfel H, Griss P. Fixation by ingrowth. In: Callaghan JJ, Rosenberg AG, Rubash HE, editors. The Adult Hip. Philadelphia: Lippincott Williams & Wilkins; 2007. pp. 195-206

[48] Hozack WJ et al. Primary cementless hip arthroplasty with a titanium plasma sprayed prosthesis. Clinical Orthopaedics and Related Research. 1996;**333**:217-225

[49] Jasty M et al. In vivo skeletal responses to porous-surfaced implants subjected to small induced motions. The Journal of Bone and Joint Surgery. 1997;**79**(5):707-714

[50] Bobyn JD et al. Characteristics of bone ingrowth and interface mechanics of a new porous tantalum biomaterial. The Journal of Bone and Joint Surgery. 1999;**81**(5):907-914

[51] McKellop H et al. Development of an extremely wear-resistant ultra high molecular weight polyethylene for total hip replacements. Journal of Orthopaedic Research. 1999;**17**(2):157-167

[52] Engh CA Jr et al. A prospective, randomized study of cross-linked and non-cross-linked polyethylene for total hip arthroplasty at 10-year follow-up. The Journal of Arthroplasty. 2012;**27**(8 Suppl):2-7.e1

[53] Schwartsmann CR et al. Novas superfícies em artroplastia total do quadril. Revista Brasileira de Ortopedia. 2012;**47**:154-159

[54] Clarke MT et al. Levels of metal ions after small- and large-diameter metal-on-metal hip arthroplasty. The Journal of Bone and Joint Surgery. 2003;**85**(6):913-917

[55] Pandit H et al. Pseudotumours associated with metal-on-metal hip resurfacings. The Journal of Bone and Joint Surgery. 2008;**90**(7):847-851

[56] Tower SS. Arthroprosthetic cobaltism: Neurological and cardiac

manifestations in two patients with metal-on-metal arthroplasty: A case report. The Journal of Bone and Joint Surgery. 2010;**92**(17):2847-2851

[57] Ladon D et al. Changes in metal levels and chromosome aberrations in the peripheral blood of patients after metal-on-metal hip arthroplasty. The Journal of Arthroplasty. 2004;**19**(8 Suppl 3):78-83

[58] Ziaee H et al. Transplacental transfer of cobalt and chromium in patients with metal-on-metal hip arthroplasty: A controlled study. The Journal of Bone and Joint Surgery. 2007;**89**(3):301-305

[59] Jarrett CA et al. The squeaking hip: A phenomenon of ceramic-on-ceramic total hip arthroplasty. The Journal of Bone and Joint Surgery. 2009;**91**(6):1344-1349

[60] Restrepo C et al. The noisy ceramic hip: Is component malpositioning the cause? The Journal of Arthroplasty. 2008;**23**(5):643-649

[61] Min BW et al. Delayed fracture of a ceramic insert with modern ceramic total hip replacement. The Journal of Arthroplasty. 2007;**22**(1):136-139

[62] Walter WL et al. Edge loading in third generation alumina ceramic-on-ceramic bearings: Stripe wear. Journal of Arthroplasty. 2004;**19**(4):402-413

[63] Canale ST, Beaty JH. Arthroplasty of the hip. In: Campbell's Operative Orthopaedics. 12th ed. 2012. Vol. I. pp. 158-310

[64] Garellick G, Rogmark C, Kärrholm J, Rolfson O. Swedish Hip Arthroplasty Register Annual Report. 2012; 113-116

[65] Australian Orthopaedic Association National Joint Replacement Registry. Annual Report. 2014—Mortality following Primary Hip and Knee Replacement. Available from: https://aoanjrr.dmac.adelaide.edu.au/documents/10180/172288/Mortality%20following%20Primary%20Hip%20and%20Knee%20Replacement

[66] American Academy of Orthopaedic Surgeons. AAOS Clinical Practice Guidelines (CPG): Preventing Venous Thromboembolic Disease in Patients Undergoing Elective Hip and Knee Arthroplasty. Available from: http://www.aaos.org/Research/guidelines/VTE/VTE_guideline.asp

[67] Johnson R, Carmichael JH, Almond HG, Loynes RP. Deep venous thrombosis following Charnley arthroplasty. Clinical Orthopaedics and Related Research. 1978;**132**:24-30

[68] American College of Chest Physicians. Antithrombotic Therapy and the Prevention of Thrombosis: American College of Chest Physicians Evidence-based Guidelines. Resources related to these guidelines can be found on the ACCP Antithrombotic Guidelines 9th Ed. 2012

[69] ISMP—Institute for Safe Medication Practices. Monitoring FDA MedWatch Reports Anticoagulants the Leading Reported Drug Risk in 2011. Available from: http://www.ismp.org/quarterwatch/pdfs/2011Q4.pdf

[70] American Academy of Orthopaedic Surgeons. AAOS Clinical Practice Guidelines (CPG): Preventing Venous Thromboembolic Disease in Patients Undergoing Elective Hip and Knee Arthroplasty. Second edition. 2011

[71] Jevsevar D, Shea K, Cummins D, Murray J, Sanders J. Recent changes in the AAOS evidence-based clinical practice guidelines process. The Journal of Bone and Joint Surgery. 2014;**96**(20):1740-1741. DOI: 10.2106/JBJS.N.00658

[72] Brooks PJ. Dislocation following total hip replacement: Causes and cures. The Bone & Joint Journal.

2013;**95-B**(11 Suppl A):67-69. DOI: 10.1302/0301-620X.95B11.32645

[73] Lindgren V, Garellick G, Kärrholm J, Wretenberg P. The type of surgical approach influences the risk of revision in total hip arthroplasty: A study from the Swedish Hip Arthroplasty Register of 90,662 total hipreplacements with 3 different cemented prostheses. Acta Orthopaedica. 2012;**83**(6):559-565. DOI: 10.3109/17453674.2012.742394

[74] Byström S, Espehaug B, Furnes O, Havelin LI, Norwegian Arthroplasty Register. Femoral head size is a risk factor for total hip luxation: A study of 42,987 primary hip arthroplasties from the Norwegian Arthroplasty Register. Acta Orthopaedica Scandinavica. 2003;**74**(5):514-524

[75] Prietzel T, Hammer N, Schleifenbaum S, Adler D, Pretzsch M, Köhler L, et al. The impact of capsular repair on the dislocation rate after primary total hip arthroplasty: A retrospective analysis of 1972 cases. Zeitschrift für Orthopädie und Unfallchirurgie. 2014;**152**(2):130-143. DOI: 10.1055/s-0034-1368209

[76] Barrack RL. Neurovascular injury: Avoiding catastrophe. The Journal of Arthroplasty. 2004;**19**(4 Suppl 1):104-107

[77] Post ZD, Orozco F, Diaz-Ledezma C, Hozack WJ, Ong A. Direct anterior approach for total hip arthroplasty: Indications, technique, and results. The Journal of the American Academy of Orthopaedic Surgeons. 2014;**22**(9):595-603

[78] Eggli S, Hankemayer S, Müller ME. Nerve palsy after leg lengthening in total replacement arthroplasty for developmental dysplasia of the hip. The Journal of Bone and Joint Surgery. 1999;**81**(5):843-845

[79] Zappe B, Glauser PM, Majewski M, Stöckli HR, Ochsner PE. Long-term prognosis of nerve palsy after total hip arthroplasty: Results of two-year-follow-ups and long-term results after a mean time of 8 years. Archives of Orthopaedic and Trauma Surgery. 2014;**134**(10):1477-1482. DOI: 10.1007/s00402-014-2038-0

[80] JH1 P, Hozack B, Kim P, Norton R, Mandel S, Restrepo C, et al. Common peroneal nerve palsy following total hip arthroplasty: Prognostic factors for recovery. The Journal of Bone and Joint Surgery. 2013;**95**(9):e551-e555. DOI: 10.2106/JBJS.L.00160

[81] Wasielewski RC, Cooperstein LA, Kruger MP, Rubash HE. Acetabular anatomy and the transacetabular fixation of screws in total hip arthroplasty. The Journal of Bone and Joint Surgery. 1990;**72**(4):501-508

[82] Masri BA, Meek RM, Duncan CP. Periprosthetic fractures evaluation and treatment. Clinical Orthopaedics and Related Research. 2004;**420**:80-95. DOI: 10.1097/00003086-200403000-00012

[83] NV1 G, Mitchell PA, Masri BA, Garbuz DS, Duncan CP. Principles of management and results of treating the fractured femur during and after total hip arthroplasty. Instructional Course Lectures. 2003;**52**:309-322

[84] Misur PN, Duncan CP, Masri BA. The treatment of periprosthetic femoral fractures after total hip arthroplasty. JBJS Reviews. 2014;**2**(8):1-9

[85] Parvizi J, Gehrke T. Proceedings of the International Consensus Meeting on Periprosthetic Joint Infection. Available from: http://www.msis-na.org/wp-content/themes/msis-temp/pdf/ism periprosthetic-joint-information.pdf

[86] Mauerhan DR, Nelson CL, Smith DL, Fitzgerald RH Jr, Slama TG, Petty RW, et al. Prophylaxis against infection in total joint arthroplasty. One day of

cefuroxime compared with three days of cefazolin. The Journal of Bone and Joint Surgery. 1994;**76**(1):39-45

[87] Klouche S, Lhotellier L, Mamoudy P. Infected total hip arthroplasty treated by an irrigation-debridement/ component retention protocol. A prospective study in a 12-case series with minimum 2 years' follow-up. Orthopaedics & Traumatology, Surgery & Research. 2011;**97**(2):134-138

[88] Espehaug B, Furnes O, Havelin LI, Engesaeter LB, Vollset SEJ. The type of cement and failure of total hip replacements. The Journal of Bone and Joint Surgery. 2002;**84**(6):832-838

[89] Garellick G, Rogmark C, Kärrholm J, Rolfson O. Swedish Hip Arthroplasty Register Annual Report. 2012

[90] National Joint Registry for England and Wales. 11th Annual Report. 2014. Available from: http://www-new.njrcentre.org.uk/njrcentre/Portals/0/Documents/England/Reports/11th_annual_report /NJR%2011th%20Annual%20Report%202014.pdf [Accessed: Jan 26, 2015]

[91] Troelsen A, Malchau E, Sillesen N, Malchau H. A review of current fixation use and registry outcomes in total hip arthroplasty: The uncemented paradox. Clinical Orthopaedics and Related Research. 2013;**471**(7):2052-2059. DOI: 10.1007/s11999-013-2941-7

[92] Wyatt M, Hooper G, Frampton C, Rothwell A. Survival outcomes of cemented compared to uncemented stems in primary total hip replacement. World Journal of Orthopedics. 2014;**5**(5): 591-596. DOI: 10.5312/wjo.v5.i5.591

[93] Australian Orthopaedic Association National Joint Replacement Registry. Annual Report. 2014. Available from: https://aoanjrr.dmac.adelaide.edu.au/documents/10180/172288/Mortality%20following%20Primary%20Hip%20and%20Knee%20Replacement [Accessed: Jan 26, 2015]

[94] McLaughlin JR, Lee KR. Uncemented total hip arthroplasty with a tapered femoral component: A 22- to 26-year follow-up study. Orthopedics. 2010;**33**(9):639. DOI: 10.3928/01477447-20100722-40

[95] Evola FR, Evola G, Graceffa A, Sessa A, Pavone V, Costarella L, et al. Performance of the CLS Spotorno uncemented stem in the third decade after implantation. The Bone & Joint Journal. 2014;**96-B**(4):455-461. DOI: 10.1302/0301-620X.96B4.32607

[96] Chawda M, Hucker P, Whitehouse SL, Crawford RW, English H, Donnelly WJ. Comparison of cemented vs uncemented acetabular component positioning using an imageless navigation system. The Journal of Arthroplasty. 2009;**24**(8):1170-1173. DOI: 10.1016/j.arth.2008.09.018

[97] Breusch SJ, Norman TL, Schneider U, Reitzel T, Blaha JD, Lukoschek M. Lavage technique in total hip arthroplasty: Jet lavage produces better cement penetration than syringe lavage in the proximal femur. The Journal of Arthroplasty. 2000;**15**(7):921-927

[98] Rolfson O. Patient-reported Outcome Measures and Health-economic Aspects of Total Hip Arthroplasty—A study of the Swedish Hip Arthroplasty Register. Institute of Clinical Sciences at Sahlgrenska Academy University of Gothenburg, Sweden. 2010

[99] Affatato S. Perspectives in Total Hip Arthroplasty: Advances in Biomaterials and their Tribological Interactions. Netherlands: Amsterdam: Elsevier: Woodhead Publishing; 2014. p. 164

[100] Pulido L, Rachala SR, Cabanela ME. Cementless acetabular revision: Past, present, and future. Revision total hip arthroplasty: The acetabular

side using cementless implants. International Orthopaedics. 2011;**35**(2):289-298

[101] Mont MA et al. The Future of high performance total hip arthroplasty. Seminars in Arthroplasty. 2006;**17**(2):88-92

[102] Galia CR et al. Caracterização físico-química de ossos liofilizados de origem bovina e humana. Revista do Colégio Brasileiro de Cirurgiões. 2009;**36**:157-160

[103] Goosen JH et al. Porous-coated femoral components with or without hydroxyapatite in primary uncemented total hip arthroplasty: A systematic review of randomized controlled trials. Archives of Orthopaedic and Trauma Surgery. 2009;**129**(9):1165-1169

[104] Walles H, Andrees-Ostovan I. VascuBone. 2013. Available from: http://www.vascubone.fraunhofer.eu/ [cited 10-11-2014]

[105] National Joint Registry for England and Wales. 11th Annual Report. 2014. Available from: http://www-new.njrcentre.org.uk/njrcentre/Portals/0/Documents/England/Reports/11th_annual_report/NJR%20 11th%20Annual%20Report%202014.pdf [Accessed: Jan 26, 2015]

[106] Hafez MA, Digioia AM. Computer-assisted total hip arthroplasty: The present and the future. Future Rheumatology. 2006;**1**(1):121-131

[107] Kunz M et al. Computer-assisted hip resurfacing using individualized drill templates. The Journal of Arthroplasty. 2010;**25**(4):600-606

[108] Sugano N et al. Comparison of mini-incision total hip arthroplasty through an anterior approach and a posterior approach using navigation. The Orthopedic Clinics of North America. 2009;**40**(3):365-370

[109] Tarwala R, Dorr LD. Robotic assisted total hip arthroplasty using the MAKO platform. Current Reviews in Musculoskeletal Medicine. 2011;**4**(3):151-156

Chapter 5

Arthroplasty as a Choice of Treatment in Hip Surgery

Mehmet Umit Cetin, Yaşar Mahsut Dincel and Yavuz Selim Kabukcuoglu

Abstract

The hip joint bears the most load in the human body. For this reason, it carries the potential risk of degenerative arthritis in individuals with a functionally active lifestyle. The main goal in the treatment of degenerative arthritis is to achieve pain relief and create a hip joint range of motion close to normal. Even today, it is not possible to transform the hip joint, which has been degenerated due to several reasons and worn out due to the physiological properties of the cartilage structure, back to its natural state. Osteotomies, resection arthroplasties and hip arthrodeses, which are designed to compensate the load distribution affecting the hip and relieve the pain, are still employed methods. Total hip arthroplasty, on the other hand, is an alternative solution for the problem. Cemented, cementless and hybrid methods are widely used for this purpose in total hip arthroplasties. The purpose of hip prosthesis surgery is to shape the bone tips and to fill the fragments with various materials and keep these two structures as separate surfaces. Total hip arthroplasty consists of a femoral component placed in the medullas of the femur and an acetabular component placed in the acetabulum. In this article we will review the aims, causes, types and techniques of total hip arthroplasty.

Keywords: acetabulum, arthritis, femur, rehabilitation, total hip arthroplasty

1. Introduction

The hip joint bears the most load in the human body. Therefore, a functional lifestyle naturally carries a potential risk of degenerative arthritis. In a hip with degenerative arthritis, the main purpose of the treatment is to relieve the pain and create a hip joint range of motion close to normal. Even today, it is not possible to transform the hip joint, which has been degenerated due to several reasons and worn out due to the physiological properties of the cartilage structure, back to its natural state.

Osteotomies, resection arthroplasties and hip arthrodeses, which are designed to compensate the load distribution affecting the hip and relieve the pain, are still employed methods. Total hip arthroplasty (THA), on the other hand, is an alternative solution for the problem. Cemented, cementless and hybrid methods are widely used for this purpose in THAs.

Three different methods, including unipolar hemiarthroplasty, bipolar hemiarthroplasty and THA can be applied in femoral neck fractures, taking the patient's age, functional status before fracture and other accompanying diseases into consideration.

Total hip arthroplasty is considered as one of the most successful orthopedic surgery methods today [1]. Ninety percent of more than 1 million THAs per year worldwide are performed for treatment of osteoarthritis. The aging world population and increasing obesity indicate that the need for THA will increase [1].

A successful joint prosthetic surgery can be achieved with clinical, functional and radiological evaluations. However, it should be noted that many other factors, such as the material used, patient's age, surgical technique and fixation method affect the results. Although hip arthroplasty can be performed successfully in many patient groups including the young ones, it should be kept in mind that young patients in particular should avoid heavy physical activities in order to prevent early failure of the prosthesis [2]. The average prosthetic survival in hip arthroplasty is 10 to 15 years. Nevertheless, there are patients who do not have complaints even after 25 years [3].

2. Total hip arthroplasty

Total hip arthroplasty consists of a femoral component placed on the medulla of the femur medulla and a component placed in the acetabulum. The cementless type of the acetabular component consists of an outer cup attached to the acetabulum and a second cup which articulates with the femoral component.

The function of the femoral component is to replace the resected femoral head and neck. As the length of the femoral neck increases, the vertical height and the medial stem-head distance also increase. In routine practice, the neck used is 8–12 mm long. The relationship between the femoral neck and implant is established based on anteversion or retroversion on the coronal plan. The vertical height of the femoral neck is measured starting from the lesser trochanter. Since the depth at which the prosthesis is placed in the femoral metaphysis to adjust the height of the vertebra is definite, the level of osteotomy is not interfered. Instead, the neck length should be adjusted.

The distance between the center of the femoral head and the stem is the medial offset distance. A wider collodiaphyseal angle shortens the moment arm of the abductors and increases limping. If this angle is narrow, the load on the stem increases and causes loosening or breakage. The vertical height of the rotation center decreases in varus hips. Accordingly, the medial offset is relatively high. The height of the greater trochanter is not an accurate indicator for the center of the head. The vertical height and medial offset in excessively varus-valgus hips are difficult to restore. Therefore, the leg length and vertical height are corrected to avoid the possibility of facing a lower extremity length discrepancy and have a biomechanically stable hip in the postoperative period [4].

Anteversion of the femoral neck is important in ensuring stability. A retroverted neck causes posterior dislocations whereas anteverted neck causes anterior dislocations. For rotational stability, the proximal part of the femoral component should fill the metaphyseal cavity completely.

The components are designed either for cemented or cementless implantations.

2.1 Cemented acetabular components

The acetabular component is thickly coated with, preferably with a layer of 6–8 mm, high-density polyethylene [5]. Stability is increased by filling cement into the vertical and horizontal grooves. Protrusions of 3-mm-high are used to increase the stability between the prosthesis and cement [5].

There are a number of factors to consider when placing the cemented acetabular components. When the acetabular component is inserted, it should maintain the normal anatomical position at 45° of inclination and 15° of anteversion. The outer surface of the acetabular component should be wrapped with at least a cement layer of 2–5 mm [6]. The boundaries of the acetabular component should be within the boundaries of the bone acetabulum.

2.2 Cemented femoral components

The most commonly used alloy is the chromium-cobalt alloy because of its high elastic modulus, which is a feature that reduces the stresses in the proximal cement layer. The medial section of the stem should be wide in the transverse section. Preferably, the lateral edge should be even wider. Thus, during compression, the load is balanced over the proximal cement mass. The onset of failure in cemented components is seen in the vicinity of the prosthetic-cement complex.

The stem should be planned to fill 80% of the transverse section of the medullary canal and the femoral component should ideally be inserted in the neutral position, in valgus position, or in varus position below 5° [7]. The risk of progressive loosening, cement fracture, proximal bone resorption is higher in patients in whom the prosthesis is inserted in varus positions above 5°. A cement layer of 2 mm thickness should be positioned 4 mm distal of the metaphyseal region of the proximal femur, and second-generation or third-generation cementing technique should be used in order to achieve the stability of the femoral component, lengthen the survival period of the implant and prevent loosening [8].

2.3 Cementing techniques

Along with the advances in surgical techniques, cementing techniques have also improved [9].

2.3.1 First-generation cementing technique

In this technique, cement is mixed manually. It is a technique that requires the least preparation of the medullary canal for prosthesis fixation. The femoral canal is opened, washed and aspirated. Cement in the dough form is applied by fingers. The prosthesis is placed manually in the neutral position (without varus or valgus). The shape of the femoral handle is sharp-edged to ensure high force transmission.

2.3.2 Second-generation cementing technique

The cement is mixed manually and applied using a "cement gun." The spongious bone in the medullary canal is removed off till the endosteal surface, and is dried after brushing and pulsatile irrigation. Plug is inserted into the medullary canal to prevent distal cement extravagation. Following the retrograde application of the cement, the prosthesis is placed in the neutral position manually or using the distal centering methods. The sharp corners of the prosthesis are rounded to increase the resistance of the cement mantle against fractures.

2.3.3 Third-generation cementing technique

In this technique, the cement is mixed in vacuum or centrifugation and applied with a cement gun. The medullary canal is cleaned to the endosteal surface. After brushing and pulsatile irrigation, the adrenaline-impregnated buffer is placed on the medulla and then dried. Cement is applied in retrograde form under pressure using a cement gun. Distal and proximal centralizers are used for the neutral placement of the prosthesis. The surfaces of the proximal and distal surfaces of the prosthesis have been treated to ensure proper load transfer to the cement.

The difference between first-generation and second-generation cementing techniques is primarily due to attempts to ameliorate the bone-cement gap. These attempts aim to avoid aseptic loosening associated with the fixation failure in the bone-cement interface resulting from fractures in the cement mantle. The third-generation cementing technique attempts to fix the cement-metal integration [10].

2.4 Cementless prosthetics

If the arthroplasty is to be long-term and durable, it is essential to maintain the mechanical balance between the prosthesis and bone surface. There are special requirements for prostheses to be integrated without cementing, which can be grouped under four sections: [11].

a. The intraosseous canal where the prosthesis is placed should be as small as possible for the press fit insertion of the prosthesis but without damaging the physiological biomechanics of bone.

b. The initial fixation of the endoprosthesis must be tight. It should reduce the likelihood of a second surgery as much as possible.

c. The design, stabilization and mechanical properties of the prosthesis must take the forces affecting the system in all directions into consideration. Some non-physiological forces may initiate bone resorption. It may even increase the risk of loosening even in cases with good primary implantation of the prosthesis.

d. The bone tissue should not be damaged during implant placement.

2.5 Fixation mechanism of the cementless total hip prostheses

Fixation is thought to happen in two stages in cementless THAs.

2.5.1 Macroscopic fixation

Also called "primary fixation," this stage of fixation aims to stabilize the prosthesis in the bone until microscopic fixation is achieved [12].

2.5.2 Microscopic fixation

Microscopic fixation is also called biological fixation. The phenomenon which means the ingrowth of the surrounding bone tissue into the prosthesis, and the trabeculation and remodeling of the bone, aims to achieve the stability of the prosthesis. In case of using a non-conforming prosthesis, the process will fail due to the resulting micro-movements. This type of fixation aims to provide bone growth directly towards the bone surface. Studies have shown that bone mineralization can develop on the titanium surface and in dependency to the porous surface configuration [12, 13]. A minimal gap of 5 micrometers (μm) is required to achieve bone growth and potential mineralized bone penetration between porous structures. This is the minimum range that allows vascularization. If the gap is between 5 and 50 μm, fibrous penetration towards the implant may be observed. Only if the gap is between 50 and 500 μm, bone penetration to the implant is possible. Therefore, the size of the pore should be between 50 and 350 μm, and preferably between 50 and

150 μm [14]. When the distance between the bone and the prosthesis is 1.5–2 mm and above, bone penetration is not sufficient due to adverse effects of micro movements. Bone penetration into the implant starts at the third week and reaches its maximum level in 6–8 weeks [15].

2.6 Response of the bone tissue to the implant

In a healthy hip, the loads passing through the joint will be transmitted distally through the femur medial cortex. While the body weight is born by the bone alone, the load is transferred to the bone through the prosthesis after THA. In this case, the point where the load is transferred from the prosthesis to the bone gains importance. The initial prosthetic designs allowed for minimal transfer of the load to the proximal medial cortex, which in turn led to stress shielding [16]. The continuity of the physiological stimulus is necessary to preserve the bone mass and prevent the development of osteoporosis. Stems with a larger diameter lead to more bone resorption than small stems [16, 17]. Bone hypertrophy is one of the results of transferring the stress load to the bone. Spongious hypertrophy in the proximal femur or cortical hypertrophy at the end or perimeter of the distal stem is observed. Therefore, distal cortical hypertrophy is not a sign of loosening, but rather the result of transferring the load from the distal to the bone [18]. Tight fit of the prosthesis at the distal and metaphyseal and distal integrations are crucial in the distribution of the loads. Optimal metaphyseal and distal integrations will significantly reduce the effects of torsional and vertical forces, and also ensure optimal transfer of the load to the bone. A tight fit of the femoral stem is necessary for a painless postoperative period. The use of porous, hydroxyapatite-coated stems, or press-fit stems, is used to achieve a rigid fixation of the proximal part of the femoral stem. Elastic fixation at the distal part is desired, thus, osteopenia in the proximal part of the femur due to lack of stimulus is avoided.

2.7 Cementless acetabular components

One of the most important advantages of THA is the successful development of cementless acetabular components. The loosening of the cemented acetabular components in elderly patients after the first decade and the loosening in young patients seen during the first decade, necessitated a revision surgery in this group [19]. Most cementless acetabular cups are porous, hemispherical cups. These cups, placed tightly in the press-fit cavities, are added projections called "pegs" and "spikes," and screws to ensure primary stability, in particular rotational stability [19].

Increasing the stability of the cups using screws ensures fast ingrowth. However, it also carries disadvantages, such as the risk of injury to the pelvic vessel and nerve, osteolysis between the screw and the cup, damage to the polyethylene surface, and screw breakage [4].

Acetabular cups, called "expansion cups", are also in use. These cups are placed in the acetabular bed by pushing and after removing the device that holds it, it springs back like a bow and holds on to the bone with the spikes on its outer surface [20].

Metal cups contain self-locking or self screwing polyethylene, produced from high-molecular-weight polyethylene. While the thickness of the metal outer cups is too thick to allow for fatigue fracture, a 5 mm thickness is recommended for the polyethylene section as it cannot meet the stress with a thickness below 5 mm. Normally, the acetabulum makes an angle of 55° with the transverse axis. The angle at which the stability of the acetabular component is best is 45°. However, placements between 35–55 and 15–20° of anteversion are considered normal. Placement of components outside these limits is predisposing conditions for forward and backward dislocations. The metal cup is placed in the acetabulum in a fashion that would better grip the superior and posterior parts [21].

2.8 Cementless femoral components

The main objective in using prostheses with a porous surface is to enable the growth of bone and its attachment to the prosthesis and achieve a biological fixation. In order for the bone to grow into the pores, primary stability of the stem during surgery and a full contact between the porous surface and live bone are required.

The shape of the porous stems, materials they are made, the location and the size of the pores show differences with each type of prosthesis. Two types of materials are used in prostheses with a porous structure. These are either made of titanium alloy, whose porous surface is made of pure, titanium fiber or made of cobalt-chromium alloy and with cobalt-chromium beads sintered to the implant. Results with both alloys have been proven to be satisfactory. However, titanium is recommended due to its high biocompatibility, high fatigue strength and low elastic modulus [22].

There are two forms of the femoral stems of the cementless porous hip prostheses; anatomic and straight. The ones with an anatomical form have a backward angulation in the metaphyseal section and a distal angulation in the distal section, in accordance with the inclination of the femoral canal. Anatomic prostheses are produced for the right and left side, with a neck properly anteverted. During the placement of anatomic prostheses, femoral medulla should be carved a little more so that the inclinations on the prosthesis can easily fit. In both types of prostheses, the aim is to fill the medullary cavity optimally, provide rotational and axial primary stability and to provide optimal load distribution by providing the broadest area of contacting surfaces between the bone and prosthesis.

The pores are generally located in the 1/3 upper metaphyseal section of the femoral component. Bone-prosthesis adhesion in the metaphyseal part ensures better absorption of the proximal loads, which in turn increases the success of long-term fixation of the stem.

The use of biologically active calcium phosphate ceramic materials has increased in recent years. Of these, tricalcium phosphate and hydroxyapatite are the most commonly used ones. These materials, which are placed as a thin layer over the surface of the prosthesis, provide a good fit to the bone and allow penetration into the bone. Hydroxyapatite provides a good osseointegration with its osteoconductive effect. The chemical structure of hydroxyapatite is similar to the bone mineral structure. It has been shown that haversian structures directly integrate with hydroxyapatite on contact surfaces with no fibrous structures, inflammatory or osteoclastic cells being observed [23].

2.9 Preoperative planning and evaluation of the patient

Preoperative planning and implant selection are of great importance in revision total hip prosthesis. The knowledge of bone stock and characteristics of the implant applied to the patient during preoperative planning and the availability of appropriate instruments and implants will increase the success of the surgery. Knowing the patient's functional status and the comorbidities before surgery will be important in drawing the limits of the intervention.

The preoperative examination starts with observation. The soft tissue surrounding the hip and the general condition of the skin is observed. Incision traces from previous surgeries are identified. Patient's gait and general posture are evaluated. The range of motion of the hip and adjacent joints, fixed or functional deformities are identified. For example, if the acetabular component is applied to the patient with excessive lordosis with standard forward and lateral angulation, insufficient tissue coverage and instability may develop following the improvement of lordosis [24]. Therefore, it should be decided whether the deformation of the lumbosacral joint is constant.

Scoliosis, poliomyelitis, developmental hip dysplasia, degenerative lumbar or thoracic disc problems and spinal fusion history should be investigated in the patient with leg length discrepancy and should be taken into account in surgical planning. The length discrepancies between the lower extremities should be determined. The "apparent length difference" is assessed by the distance measured from the umbilicus to the medial malleoli. With the blocks placed under the short leg, the pelvis is balanced and the "functional length difference" is determined. The "actual length difference" is measured by the distance between the anterior superior iliac spine on both sides and the medial malleolus. This is the most reliable clinical method, however, the method provides different according to the position of the extremity or pelvis when contracture is present [25]. Especially in the extremity where deformities such as knee contracture are present, the most definitive diagnosis method in determining the length difference is computed tomography (CT) in which the femur and tibia lengths can be measured separately [26].

For a successful surgical planning, the condition of the extremities and the joints which will not be operated should be also investigated during physical examination [27].

Direct radiographs to be taken preoperatively include the full pelvic anteroposterior (AP) radiograph focused on the symphysis pubis and full AP and lateral radiographs focused on the center of the affected hip. The pelvic radiograph is used to assess the length difference between the affected and contralateral hip joints. In particular, the structure of the femur and acetabulum are examined on hip radiographs. AP radiographs are taken in the supine position and, if possible, with the leg internally rotated at 15°. Thus, the full AP image and the actual offset of the femur with an anteverted neck at 15° are obtained. If internal rotation of the hip is not possible due to pathology, the other hip is used for evaluation [28]. Lateral radiographs are used to determine the anatomy of the femoral canal and its association with the piriformis fossa [29].

Rheumatoid arthritis, ankylosing spondylitis, Paget's disease or metabolic diseases weaken the subchondral bone and therefore the center of motion shift towards medial in case of acetabular protrusion. Lateralization of the hip's center of motion, preparation of the allograft for reconstruction of the cavity which may occur in the medial area or the necessary tools to remove the femoral head should be planned before surgery.

The femur may shift towards the superolateral due to acetabular insufficiency in hips with dysplasia. As the actual acetabulum may be smaller than normal and have inadequate bone stock, preoperative preparations may avoid potential problems in these patients. Keeping the hip center high may be an option when reconstructing the acetabulum. If the hip center is preferred to be lowered to the anatomical level of the acetabulum, acetabular components with a small diameter (40–42–44 mm) and with a fitting head and stem should be prepared. In addition, the femoral head obtained after osteotomy can be used to support the superior of the acetabulum to provide full coverage in the actual acetabulum. Another important problem that may be encountered when lowering the acetabulum to its actual position will be the vascular and nerve problems that may develop as a result of prolongation of the extremity. In particular, an elongation of more than 2.5 cm may require femoral osteotomy as it increases the potential risk [30].

2.10 Indications for total hip arthroplasty

Total hip arthroplasty is an irreversible, radical decision in hip-related diseases. Total hip prosthesis is generally recommended in two cases. The first is the presence of a chronic disease in the hip joint, which is often associated with pain and functional limitation. Degenerative and inflammatory-based diseases of the hip joint can be evaluated in this group. They can show a fast or slow progress. In addition to leg length discrepancy, limping, pelvic imbalance and related spine problems can be observed. The latter are the conditions that cause bone defects such as hip fractures, pseudoarthroses and peripheral tumors [31].

The most important finding for the decision of THA is pain. Before recommending the patient THA, a major surgery of the hip, all conservative methods such as weight loss, analgesic treatment, reducing the level of activity on a reasonable scale, choosing a job that requires less activity than a physically active job, and walking cane should be tried. These methods usually reduce the patient's complaints. Ultimately, either surgical treatment becomes unnecessary or surgery is delayed for a long period [32].

If the patient continues to experience pain in daily works, walks shorter distances, has pain despite analgesics and the changes in activities, and experiences nocturnal pain in particular despite all conservative treatment methods, THA is indicated [33].

2.11 Contraindications for total hip arthroplasty

The success of THA relies on careful patient selection and deciding the ones fit and unfit for THA. THA is a major surgical intervention in which important complications can develop and the mortality rate varies between 1 and 2% [34, 35]. For this reason, when THA is indicated, the patient should be evaluated carefully regarding the presence of systemic diseases which will not allow for a major surgery. Therefore, the necessary consultation of the patient should be performed in the postoperative period. It should be kept in mind that some patients may have cardiopulmonary, metabolic, genitourinary and liver problems, hypertension, or hidden malignancies that need to be corrected before major surgical intervention.

Definite contraindications for THA include; the presence of an active infection in the hips or other areas outside the hip, and the presence of systemic diseases which will significantly increase the morbidity or mortality rate of the patient [36]. Charcot joint, loss of abductor muscles, rapidly progressive neurological diseases, dementia and successful hip arthrodesis are reported to be relatively contraindicated [37].

3. Surgical approaches

When performing hip arthroplasty, the ideal surgical approach should provide adequate space for the femoral neck incision, head removal and access to the acetabulum while keeping the damage to muscle functions at minimum. Surgical approaches may vary based on whether the patient is lying on his back or side, having had a greater trochanter bone incision and whether the hip is pulled forwards or backwards. The most commonly used approaches in hip arthroplasties are; anterior, anterolateral, lateral, posterior and posterolateral approaches. Each surgical approach has several advantages and difficulties. There is no ideal implant model or system that will fit and be used easily in every situation for each patient. For this reason, the surgeon must have a general knowledge about the design of the prosthetic elements, and about its weaknesses and strengths. Implant selection should be made by taking the patient's needs, the time the implant should survive, the patient's activity level, the quality and size of the bone, the implants and surgical instruments available and of course the surgeon's experience into account.

3.1 Anterolateral approach

The greatest advantage of this procedure is that the patient lies in the supine position. Thus, orientation of the patient is easier, the length of the leg is easier to evaluate during surgery and the appearance of the acetabulum is much neater [38]. Lower dislocation rates have been reported with this approach [39, 40]. The major disadvantage of the approach is the damage to the gluteus medius localized at the anterior of the greater trochanter and damage to the superior gluteal nerve located 5 cm proximal of the greater trochanter, which may lead to limping [41].

3.2 Direct lateral approach

This approach has a lower dislocation rate compared to the posterior approach [42, 43]. While lower rates of neurological complications have been reported compared to the anterolateral approach, it has been shown that the rate of limping due to gluteus medius injury is higher than the posterior approach [44]. In the lateral approach, the splitting of the gluteus medius starting from the upper end of the greater trochanter major to 6 cm towards the proximal puts superior gluteal nerve at risk, thus, caution should be exercised [45].

3.3 Posterior approach

It is a safe method to reach the hip joint easily and quickly. The main advantages of this approach are that it does not damage the abductor mechanism, does not impair the functionality of the iliotibial band, and it allows for rapid rehabilitation in the postoperative period. In this approach, while retraction is more comfortable, orientation of the patient is more difficult. Compared to the anterolateral approach, there is less bleeding and better preservation of the abductor muscle strength, however, higher hip dislocation rates have been reported [46, 47]. In addition, in case of failing to pay due attention, the risk of damage to the sciatic nerve is high with this approach [48].

4. Rehabilitation

Following THAs, most of the patients experience some functional deficits and disorders non-concurrent with pain. Muscle weaknesses and muscle atrophies may be permanent. Asymmetrical extremity loading in functional activities and Trendelenburg gait due to the weakness of the abductor muscles of the hip are the most common problems. Functional disorders can lead to a decrease in mobility and physical activity, and dependency in daily life. Therefore, the rehabilitation of the patients after surgery is crucial.

In THAs, the rehabilitation process should begin with preoperative evaluation, followed by training and rehabilitation. An early and intensive rehabilitation program should be applied to reduce early muscle strength and function loss after THA. The postoperative rehabilitation program includes prevention of complications, reeducation of the muscles, strengthening and flexibility exercises, gait and balance training, functional exercises and home exercises. In order to prevent complications, patients should be trained about dislocation positions immediately after the surgery and precautions should be taken during their mobilization. Early rehabilitation includes active ankle pump, gait training, low impact isometric exercises, and isotonic exercises for hip abductors, extensors and knee extensors. If cemented THA was performed, full weight-bearing is allowed with the use of double crutches. For cementless THA patients, walking with aids or partial weight-bearing is allowed for 6 weeks. This program can be extended until the 12th week [49].

The use of aquatic therapy to stimulate early healing, low-frequency electrical stimulation to strengthen the weak muscles, and biofeedback to alter the load distribution provide additional benefits [50].

The exercise program in the late term consists of eight exercise groups, focusing on functional tasks, activities of daily living, balance, strength, endurance and cardiovascular fitness. In order to ensure cardiovascular compliance, patients are directed to non-stressful sports and exercises.

Arthroplasty techniques and the rehabilitation programs associated with them have improved in recent years [51].

5. Complications

5.1 Complications during surgery

The worst operative complication recorded in the literature is the main iliac vein rupture following the perforation of the medial wall during acetabular reaming [52]. The same complication has also been reported during the screwing of the acetabular cups of some cemented and cementless prostheses [53].

Another important complication observed is nerve lesion. The prevalence rate varies between 0.7 and 3.5% in primary arthroplasty and may go up to 7.5% in revisions [53].

Another complication, femoral shaft fractures is easier to avoid than to treat. Fitzgerald et al. reported a 17.6% rate of fracture during cementless hip arthroplasty and a rate of 3.5% in revision surgeries [54].

5.2 Early-term postoperative complications

Since hematoma lays a suitable ground for infection, which is one of the most important and feared complications of THA, it is necessary to pay attention to hemostasis during surgery. The main part of the treatment is to prevent secondary infection of hematoma.

Previous hip surgery or revision total hip replacement, posterior surgical approach, incorrect positioning of one or both of the components, femur catching the pelvis or residual osteophytes, wedging of the neck of the femoral component to the edge of the acetabular component, inadequate soft tissue balancing, insufficiency or weakness of the abductor muscle group, avulsion or pseudoarthrosis of the greater trochanter, incompatibility or improper positioning in the perioperative period are the factors that cause dislocation. In the literature, the incidence of dislocation following THA has been reported to vary between 1 and 3%. There is a higher risk of dislocation in revision surgeries compared to primary surgeries [55].

Infection may develop 3 months after THA. These infections are classified as deep and superficial infections. Those who do not penetrate through the fascia are called “superficial” and those who penetrate beyond the fascia are called “deep” infections [56]. The incidence of the infections varies between 0.4 and 3% [57].

Thromboembolism and pulmonary embolism are the most serious complications seen after THA. It is the most common cause of death in the first three postoperative months and is responsible for 50% of the postoperative mortality following THA [58].

5.3 Late-term postoperative complications

Unceasing and unexplained pain that continues from surgery indicates an infection with a slow course. In general, pain is present both at rest and during active weight-bearing. Deep infections in the late term necessitates the removal of the implants in almost all patients.

Heterotopic ossification has an incidence rate of 3–5%. Ankylosing spondylitis is more common in cases with previous posttraumatic arthritis, hypertrophic osteoarthritis and heterotopic ossification [59].

6. Conclusion

Total hip arthroplasty is a surgery performed to provide painless movement of the hip joint and to gain the muscles, ligaments and other soft tissue that control the joint functionality. Hip arthroplasty is a surgical method with very successful results and performed in the presence of pain due to hip arthritis, avascular necrosis, ankylosing spondylitis and the proximal end fractures of the femur.

Total hip arthroplasty is a surgical treatment modality successful in eliminating the hip problems that cannot be solved with medical treatments and has an increasing worldwide popularity. But it should be kept in mind that this success of THA relies on proper patient selection, precise planning before surgery, selection of an implant compatible with the indication, and implementation of an effective rehabilitation program following surgery.

Author details

Mehmet Umit Cetin, Yaşar Mahsut Dincel* and Yavuz Selim Kabukcuoglu
Department of Orthopedics and Traumatology, Faculty of Medicine, Namık Kemal University, Tekirdag, Turkey

*Address all correspondence to: ymd61@hotmail.com

References

[1] Pivec R, Johnson AJ, Mears SC, Mont MA. Hip arthroplasty. Lancet. 2012;**380**:1768-1777

[2] Crowther JD, Lachiewicz PF. Survival and polyethylene wear of porous-coated acetabular components in patients less than fifty years old: Results at nine to fourteen years. The Journal of Bone and Joint Surgery. American Volume. 2002;**84-A**:729-735

[3] Caton J, Prudhon JL. Over 25 years survival after Charnley's total hip arthroplasty. International Orthopaedics. 2011;**35**:185-188

[4] Harkess JW, Crockarell JR. Arthroplasty of the hip. In: Canale ST, editor. Campbell's Operative Orthopedics. Vol. 1. Philadelphia, PA: Mosby; 2008. pp. 312-481

[5] Savory CG, Hamilton WG, Engh CA, Valle CJD, Rosenberg AG, Galante JO. Hip designs. In: Barrack RL, Booth RE, Lonner JH, editors. Orthopaedic Knowledge Update: Hip and Knee Reconstruction. 3rd ed. Rosemont, Illionis: American Academy of Orthopaedic Surgeons; 2006. pp. 345-368

[6] Bilgen MS, Özdel A, Bilge ÖF. Design and application techniques of acetabular components [Article in Turkish]. Totbid Journal. 2013;**12**:225-238

[7] Callaghan JJ, Bracha P, Liu SS, Piyaworakhun S, Goetz DD, Johnston RC. Survivorship of a Charnley total hip arthroplasty. A concise follow-up, at a minimum of thirty-five years, of previous reports. The Journal of Bone and Joint Surgery. American Volume. 2009;**91**:2617-2621

[8] Beksaç B, Özden VE, Tözün İR. Properties of the femoral components in total hip arthroplasty [Article in Turkish]. Totbid Journal. 2013;**12**:215-218

[9] Wang Y, Han P, Gu W, Shi Z, Li D, Wang C. Cement oscillation increases interlock strength at the cement-bone interface, with commentary. Orthopedics. 2009;**32**:325

[10] Akman S, Seçkiner M, Öztürk F. Biomaterials in orthopedics and traumatology [Article in Turkish]. Totbid Journal. 2005;**1**:38-39

[11] Morscher EW. Cementless total hip arthroplasty. Clinical Orthopaedics and Related Research. 1983;**181**:76-91

[12] Crowninshield R. An overview of prosthetic materials for fixation. Clinical Orthopaedics and Related Research. 1988;**235**:166-172

[13] McCutchen JW, Collier JP, Mayor MB. Osseointegration of titanium implants in total hip arthroplasty. Clinical Orthopaedics and Related Research. 1990;**261**:114-125

[14] McPherson EJ. Adult reconstruction. In: Miller DM, editor. Review of Orthopaedics. Philadelphia, PA: WB Saunders Company; 2004. pp. 266-308

[15] Haddad RJ Jr, Cook SD, Thomas KA. Biological fixation of porous-coated implants. The Journal of Bone and Joint Surgery. American Volume. 1987;**69**:1459-1466

[16] Engh CA, Bobyn JD. The influence of stem size and extent of porous coating on femoral bone resorption after primary cementless hip arthroplasty. Clinical Orthopaedics and Related Research. 1988;**231**:7-28

[17] Lewis JL, Askew MJ, Wixson RL, Kramer GM, Tarr RR. The influence of prosthetic stem stiffness and of a calcar collar on stresses in the proximal end of the femur with a cemented femoral component. The Journal of Bone and Joint Surgery. American Volume. 1984;**66**:280-286

[18] Sumner DR, Galante JO. Determinants of stress shielding: Design versus materials versus interface. Clinical Orthopaedics and Related Research. 1992;**274**:202-212

[19] Harris WH. Results of uncemented cups: A critical appraisal at 15 years. Clinical Orthopaedics and Related Research. 2003;**417**:121-125

[20] Pagnano W, Hanssen AD, Lewallen DG, Shaughnessy WJ. The effect of superior placement of the acetabular component on the rate of loosening after total hip arthroplasty. The Journal of Bone and Joint Surgery. American Volume. 1996;**78**:1004-1014

[21] DiFazio F, Shon WY, Salvati EA, Wilson PD Jr. Long-term results of total hip arthroplasty with a cemented custom-designed swan-neck femoral component for congenital dislocation or severe dysplasia: A follow-up note. The Journal of Bone and Joint Surgery. American Volume. 2002;**84-A**:204-207

[22] Papagelopoulos PJ, Trousdale RT, Lewallen DG. Total hip arthroplasty with femoral osteotomy for proximal femoral deformity. Clinical Orthopaedics and Related Research. 1996;**332**:151-162

[23] Cook SD, Thomas KA, Kay FJ, Jarcho M. Hydroxyapatite-coated porous titanium for use as an orthopedic biologic attachments system. Clinical Orthopaedics and Related Research. 1988;**230**:303-312

[24] Aufranc OE, Aufranc ST. Evaluation of the patient with an arthritic hip. In: Stillwell WT, editor. The Art of Total Hip Arthroplasty. Orlando, FL: Grune & Stratton; 1987. pp. 123-132

[25] Beattie P, Isaacson K, Riddle DL, Rothstein JM. Validity of derived measurements of leg-length differences obtained by use of a tape measure. Physical Therapy. 1990;**70**:150-157

[26] Aaron A, Weinstein D, Thickman D, Eilert R. Comparison of orthoroentgenography and computed tomography in the measurement of limb-length discrepancy. The Journal of Bone and Joint Surgery. American Volume. 1992;**74**:897-902

[27] Özden VE, Beksaç B, Tözün İR. Preoperative planning and its significance [Article in Turkish]. Totbid Journal. 2013;**12**:207-214

[28] D'Antonio JA. Preoperative templating and choosing the implant for primary THA in the young patient. Instructional Course Lectures. 1994;**43**:339-346

[29] Crawford RW, Psychoyios V, Gie G, Ling R, Murray D. Incomplete cement mantles in the sagittal femoral plane: An anatomical explanation. Acta Orthopaedica Scandinavica. 1999;**70**:596-598

[30] Jasty M, Anderson MJ, Harris WH. Total hip replacement for developmental dysplasia of the hip. Clinical Orthopaedics and Related Research. 1995;**311**:40-45

[31] Temelli Y, Kılıçoğlu Ö. Total kalça protezinde hasta seçimi ve zamanlama. In: Yazıcıoğlu Ö, Salvati EA, Göksan SB, Kılıçoğlu Ö, editors. Total Kalça Artroplastisi. 1st ed. İstanbul: Ekin Yayıncılık; 2009. pp. 116-122

[32] Azboy İ, Demirtaş A, Uçar BY. Indications for total hip arthroplasty and patient selection [Article in Turkish]. Totbid Journal. 2013;**12**:201-206

[33] Saleh A, Faour M, Sultan AA, Brigati DP, Molloy RM, Mont MA. Emergency department visits within thirty days of discharge after primary total hip arthroplasty: A hidden quality measure. The Journal of Arthroplasty. 2018. pii: S0883-5403(18)30736-8. DOI: 10.1016/j.arth.2018.08.032 [Epub ahead of print]

[34] Thompson R, Kane RL, Gromala T, McLaughlin B, Flood S, Morris N, et al. Complications and short-term outcomes associated with total hip arthroplasty in teaching and community hospitals. The Journal of Arthroplasty. 2002;**17**:32-40

[35] Poultsides LA, Ma Y, Della Valle AG, Chiu YL, Sculco TP, Memtsoudis SG. In-hospital surgical site infections after primary hip and knee arthroplasty—Incidence and risk factors. The Journal of Arthroplasty. 2013;**28**:385-389

[36] Guo EW, Sayeed Z, Padela MT, Qazi M, Zekaj M, Schaefer P, et al. Improving total joint replacement with continuous quality improvement methods and tools. The Orthopedic Clinics of North America. 2018;**49**:397-403

[37] Kuijpers MFL, Hannink G, van Steenbergen LN, Schreurs BW. Total hip arthroplasty in young patients in The Netherlands: Trend analysis of >19,000 primary hip replacements in the Dutch arthroplasty register. The Journal of Arthroplasty. 2018. pii: S0883-5403(18)30724-1. DOI: 10.1016/j.arth.2018.08.020 [Epub ahead of print]

[38] Ritter MA, Harty LD, Keating ME, Faris PM, Meding JB. A clinical comparison of the anterolateral and posterolateral approaches to the hip. Clinical Orthopaedics and Related Research. 2001;**385**:95-99

[39] Mallory TH, Lombardi AV Jr, Fada RA, Herrington SM, Eberle RW. Dislocation after total hip arthroplasty using the anterolateral abductor split approach. Clinical Orthopaedics and Related Research. 1999;**358**:166-172

[40] McCollum DE, Gray WJ. Dislocation after total hip arthroplasty. Causes and prevention. Clinical Orthopaedics and Related Research. 1990;**261**:159-170

[41] Baker AS, Bitounis VC. Abductor function after total hip replacement. An electromyographic and clinical review. Journal of Bone and Joint Surgery. British Volume (London). 1989;**71-B**:47-50

[42] DeLee JG, Charnley J. Radiological demarcation of cemented sockets in total hip replacement. Clinical Orthopaedics and Related Research. 1976;**121**:20-32

[43] Frndak PA, Mallory TH, Lombardi AV Jr. Translateral surgical approach to the hip. The abductor muscle "split". Clinical Orthopaedics and Related Research. 1993;**295**:135-141

[44] Van der Linde MJ, Tonino AJ. Nerve injury after hip arthroplasty. 5/600 cases after uncemented hip replacement, anterolateral approach versus direct lateral approach. Acta Orthopaedica Scandinavica. 1997;**68**:521-523

[45] Jacobs LG, Buxton RA. The course of the superior gluteal nerve in the lateral approach to the hip. The Journal of Bone and Joint Surgery. American Volume. 1989;**71-A**:1239-1243

[46] Weale AE, Newman P, Ferguson IT, Bannister GC. Nerve injury after posterior and direct lateral approaches for hip replacement. A clinical and electrophysiological study. Journal of Bone and Joint Surgery. British Volume (London). 1996;**78**:899-902

[47] Roberts JM, Fu FH, McClain EJ, Ferguson AB Jr. A comparison of the posterolateral and anterolateral approaches to total hip arthroplasty. Clinical Orthopaedics and Related Research. 1984;**187**:205-210

[48] Dayıcan A, Özkan G, Tümöz MA. Nerve injuries in total hip arthroplasty and protection [Article in Turkish]. Totbid Journal. 2004;**3**:3-4

[49] Ribinik P, Le Moine F, de Korvin G, Coudeyre E, Genty M, Rannou F, et al. Physical and rehabilitation medicine (PRM) care pathways: "Patients after total hip arthroplasty". Annals of Physical and Rehabilitation Medicine. 2012;**55**:540-545

[50] Pataky Z, De León Rodriguez D, Golay A, Assal M, Assal JP, Hauert CA. Biofeedback training for partial weight bearing in patients after total hip arthroplasty. Archives of Physical Medicine and Rehabilitation. 2009;**90**:1435-1438

[51] Can F. Total hip arthroplasty, rehabilitation [Article in Turkish]. Totbid Journal. 2013;**12**:292-308

[52] Mallory TH. Rupture of the common iliac vein from reaming the acetabulum during total hip replacement. A case report. The Journal of Bone and Joint Surgery. American Volume. 1972;**54**:276-277

[53] Keating ME, Ritter MA, Faris PM. Structures at risk from medially placed acetabular screw. The Journal of Bone and Joint Surgery. American Volume. 1990;**72**:509-511

[54] Fitzgerald RH Jr, Brindley GW, Kavanagh BF. The uncemented total hip arthroplasty. Intraoperative femoral fractures. Clinical Orthopaedics and Related Research. 1988;**235**:61-66

[55] Dorr LD, Wolf AW, Chandler R, Conaty JP. Classification and treatment of dislocations of total hip arthroplasty. Clinical Orthopaedics and Related Research. 1983;**173**:151-158

[56] Fitzgerald RH Jr. Total hip arthroplasty sepsis. Prevention and diagnosis. The Orthopedic Clinics of North America. 1992;**23**:259-264

[57] Tsukayama DT, Estrada R, Gustilo RB. Infection after total hip arthroplasty. A study of treatment of one hundred and six infections. The Journal of Bone and Joint Surgery. American Volume. 1996;**78**:512-523

[58] Planès A, Vochelle N, Fagola M, Feret J, Bellaud M. Prevention of deep vein thrombosis after total hip replacement. The effect of low-molecular-weight heparin with spinal and general anaesthesia. Journal of Bone and Joint Surgery. British Volume (London). 1991;**73**:418-422

[59] Nilsson OS, Persson PE. Heterotopic bone formation after joint replacement. Current Opinion in Rheumatology. 1999;**11**:127-131